Deceived

CLAUDIA BLACK

Deceived
Facing the Trauma
of Sexual Betrayal

CENTRAL RECOVERY PRESS

LAS VEGAS

Central Recovery Press (CRP) is committed to publishing exceptional materials addressing addiction treatment, recovery, and behavioral healthcare topics.

For more information, visit www.centralrecoverypress.com.

Publisher: Central Recovery Press
             3321 N. Buffalo Drive
             Las Vegas, NV 89129

24 23 22 21 20 19   1 2 3 4 5

Library of Congress Cataloging-in-Publication Data
Names: Black, Claudia, author.
Title: Deceived : facing the traumas of sexual betrayal / Claudia Black.
Description: Revised and updated edition. | Las Vegas : Central Recovery
   Press, [2019] | Revised edition of the author's Deceived, 2009. | Includes
   bibliographical references.
Identifiers: LCCN 2019006210 (print) | LCCN 2019013343 (ebook) | ISBN
   9781949481099 (ebook) | ISBN 9781949481082 (pbk. : alk. paper)
Subjects: LCSH: Women--Psychology. | Men--Sexual behavior. |
   Betrayal--Psychological aspects. | Adultery--Psychological aspects.
Classification: LCC HQ1206 (ebook) | LCC HQ1206 .B445 2019 (print) | DDC
   646.7/8--dc23
LC record available at https://lccn.loc.gov/2019006210

Photo of Claudia Black by Winifred Whitfield. Used with permission.

Publisher's Note:
This book contains general information about sex addiction and its effects on relationships. The information is not medical advice. This book is not an alternative to medical advice from your doctor or other professional healthcare provider.

Our books represent the experiences and opinions of their authors only. Every effort has been made to ensure that events, institutions, and statistics presented in our books as facts are accurate and up-to-date. To protect their privacy, the names of some of the people, places, and institutions in this book may have been changed.

Cover design and interior by Sara Streifel, Think Creative Design.

To the Women of the Lodge

*Those who have entered the doors and begun their
healing and those yet to come*

May You Soar

Contents

Preface

To live with sexual betrayal is to live with deceit. *Deception* means to cause a person to believe what is not true, to mislead, betray, delude, or dupe. When your partner is engaging in sexual behavior that violates the values of your relationship, he will go to great lengths to conceal his behavior. In that process, his deception involves falsehood or the deliberate concealment or misrepresentation of truth.

To *mislead* means to lead into error, but not invariably with the intent to harm. His behavior is not intentionally meant to harm you. More likely than not he has deluded himself by believing you will never know, and if you don't know, you will not be hurt.

To *betray* implies a faithlessness that brings another to a disadvantage or into danger. This faithlessness puts your relationship on an unequal playing field. Instead of an equal partnership, you are set up for a "one up" and "one down" relationship, with you being the "one down." Without honesty, your relationship is based on an illusion. While betrayal puts your relationship in jeopardy, it can also create physical danger for you with unsafe sex practices and/or the rage that comes from jilted lovers.

To *delude* is to mislead to the point of rendering another unable to detect a falsehood or make sound judgment. Your partner, as if a magician, has become a master of deception.

To *dupe* means to delude another by playing upon that person's susceptibility or naiveté. Time after time your partner has relied on your naiveté, your need to want to believe him, and your fears of what it means to know the truth.

To live like this is traumatic to your whole being.

✳ ✳ ✳

When *Deceived* was first published in 2009, it was one of the first books to speak to female partners of men who were acting out sexually in an addictive manner. At that time, the language within the professional field of those working with the addicted and their partners emanated from an addiction model. While I and other early pioneers were addressing the trauma of betrayal, we did not have the language and depth of knowledge about trauma responses that have more recently been validating and critical to the partner in his or her healing. In the past few years the emphasis for healing and recovery is much more steeped in treatment that acknowledges and responds to the traumatic stress and betrayal of trust experienced by partners.

This trauma and betrayal experience is now reflected in the new subtitle for *Deceived: Facing the Trauma of Sexual Betrayal.* You have been deceived, time and time again, and that is traumatic to your very being. And while you are addressing the lies and secrecy that come with deception, the impact of the trauma needs to be validated and articulated. The words "trauma" and "betrayal" afford that, therefore, in this edition, I will incorporate more knowledge about trauma and trauma responses as well as changing language so that it can enhance and acknowledge the partners' recovery process.

As the trauma lens has been incorporated into the treatment for partners, the phenomena of one's codependency has been challenged. Yet as you read, you will see that some of the women in this book, while recognizing their trauma, also find value in their understanding of codependency. In lieu of choosing an either/ or framework, they recognize that what has occurred in their relationship has been traumatic and, for some, not all, prior to the trauma of sexual deception, they engaged in what was previously considered codependent behavior and thinking. When referring to their codependent behavior, they are referring to self-defeating behaviors they learned growing up with addiction, abuse, or an otherwise impaired family system. These behaviors included discounting their own needs, learning to not show feelings, or to not trust others. It basically says you learned certain traits as a part of your survival growing up. It was what you did to bring safety and security to your life. But to continue these behaviors in adulthood only interferes with healthy self-care and the ability to be healthy in a relationship. With that meaning, this phraseology is validating.

In my book, *Unspoken Legacy: Addressing the Impact of Trauma and Addiction within the Family*, published in 2018, I reframe what was learned in a troubled family as being traumatic and much of what has been identified to be codependent is in fact a trauma response. What makes the early life experiences often traumatic is that you are subject to chronically hurtful experiences at the time in your life when you are developing your sense of worth and identity.

In *Deceived* I follow the stories of six women who worked together in a recovery group. They came to feel such power in community that they called themselves the Women of the Lodge. A handful of years later they are no longer together as a group, but continue in their recovery in various communities. I chose these particular stories as collectively they address the many variations of possible scenarios. You will also read the words of other unnamed partners and at times the words of the addict.

In my work with these women I saw them grapple with self-esteem, self-worth, and dignity at a level I had never before encountered. Was this because of the particular women I worked with? Possibly, but I think not. I think the nature of betrayal they experienced and their profound personal histories, coupled with the safety they felt in the group to claim their voices, allowed them to be authentic with each other and be true to themselves. All of these women came together as a force, and they soared. In their anguish, they cried and they were angry—oh so angry. They laughed and they loved; they bolstered one another; they laughed some more. They came to love and support each other in ways they had never previously expressed or experienced. The common denominator was simply that they each had a partner who was acting out sexually. Some of them had partners who became strong in recovery; others had partners who were never serious about recovery. Whatever their individual circumstances, some women stayed in their relationships, some ended up leaving, and some went through a divorce they did not seek. But each moved forward in her life and benefited greatly through the community of others she found in her healing process. As I continue to meet partners today, I see the same pain, the same strengths, and the same desire to find safety to be able to make decisions about their life and to move forward.

While these women had partners who did pursue treatment that may not be true in your situation. Whether or not he is willing to get help you are left with the trauma of the betrayal. Nonetheless, you can get help on your own. Your healing, which may be about trusting your gut, your self care, and boundary setting, can begin.

✳ ✳ ✳

Today more men, both heterosexual and gay, and more lesbian partners are identifying their partner as a sex addict. In this book it is not feasible to discuss the nuances and differences in the many types of relationships, but betrayal is betrayal, and we are all human. People want honesty; they want fidelity. They want trust. While I have only used heterosexual female voices, my hope is that others will find pearls in the humanness of this difficult experience.

Everyone's story is unique and you may not see your exact circumstances but my hope is that you will nonetheless feel both validation and a sense of hope from which you can garner a life that will move you forward.

As you read through *Deceived*, I encourage you to take a pen, pencil, or better yet, a marker and highlight that which speaks to you. It doesn't have to describe an exact experience but rather something about it that resonates with you. It may describe you, validate you, it may be a message you want to hang onto. It is quite likely you will have a very marked up book by the conclusion, and it is a good way to use the book as a reminder of what you need to hear again after you have completed the first read. Also, because this book is so personal and therefore can be emotional, having underlined or marked areas that are more specific to you makes it easier to access the content you want to maintain.

Writing can be a wonderful form of self-therapy, and I encourage you to journal throughout the time you are reading this book and journal in response to the questions posed at the end of each chapter. As you read and journal, remember to keep breathing. Stop periodically and reorient. Take some deep breaths. Look around your environment. What do you see? What do you hear? What do you smell? What are you touching? Do you need to take a break? What would be a healthy way to support or nurture yourself?

In reading *Deceived* it is my hope that you will better understand what is happening in your life, and find a path that offers you clarity, direction, and voice. I am honored to be a part of your journey. I remain humbled at the courage, bravery, strength, and resiliency of both female and male partners, and I continue to be in awe of the spirit of those who feel so fragile, so vulnerable, yet are so strong. As I have said many times, I cannot promise you your relationship, but I can promise you your integrity and self-respect in your personal recovery.

It's not an easy journey but it is one of profound transformation.

Acknowledgments

My heart is full when I think of all the people whose lives came together in a manner that influenced my writing this book. The first edition of *Deceived* was inspired by the many women who were part of my work with Patrick Carnes, Ralph Earle, and Diane Dillon. I was invited to lead my first group with female partners of sex addicts and that experience became a professional and personal gift for which I will always be grateful. To Diane Dillon, my co-therapist of many years in working with these women, thank you. it was an exhilarating, challenging experience of great joy, humility, and incredible teamwork in an untapped area of psychotherapy. You are a colleague from whom I learned a lot and a dear friend, and because of your insistence, I wrote this book.

For over six years, women came to group; some stayed for several years, some participated briefly, and others only paid a visit. I witnessed raw emotion, incredible courage, and triumphant transformation, and I will always carry the experiences of shared tears, laughter, touch, and love. I cherish our time together and hold you all forever in my heart. Since then I have been blessed to meet with partners attending the Intimate Treason workshop at Rio

Retreat Center at The Meadows. From all, I continue to learn about the trauma of sexual betrayal, the pain, and the recovery.

Thanks to all the women and men, named and unnamed, who shared their stories for this book and trusted me to honor the lives of others through your experiences. Your contributions are inspiring. I would like to recognize my wonderful group of women friends and my sister, Jana. I have needed you and each one of you has been with me in spirit wherever my personal and professional journey has taken me.

While there are many fine leaders within the field of addictions and sex addiction, I would like to acknowledge the pioneering work of Patrick Carnes and Jennifer Schneider who wrote the seminal books about the issues of sex addiction, sex addicts and their partners, and offered a foundational framework for work in this field; the Association of Partners of Sex Addicts Trauma Specialists (APSATS), that has further shaped the clinical work with partners through the lens of trauma; and Stefanie Carnes a leading beacon in the training of professionals working with the addict and a champion for the partners. Today there is a much stronger understanding among therapists that the partner is as deserving of resources as the person who is acting out sexually.

Thanks to my longtime assistant, Sandi Klein, who was there for the first edition and now the second. Jeri Nilson, your conceptual feedback was invaluable. You asked tough questions and prompted me for more. You embraced the stories of the female partners in a manner that allows this book to speak to even greater numbers of women. Jean Collins, Maureen Canning, and Maria C., who took the time to offer me very specific feedback for which I am most grateful. A special thank you to Cara Tripodi, coauthor of *Intimate Treason*, as we took that clinical step of recognizing the traumatic stress endured by partners. And thank you Central Recovery Press for valuing the need for materials to embrace the partners' experience.

Lastly, I lovingly acknowledge Jack Fahey, my husband of thirty-nine years. Jack was passionate about everyone's recovery. The release of this second edition of *Deceived* marks the second anniversary of his passing. Jack always believed in me and my work. He will forever be my greatest champion.

To all who pick up this book, I hope you find a path that leads to greater happiness.

CHAPTER ONE

You Are Not Alone

Why me? How could he?

Doesn't he love me? What should I do?

How can I keep this secret without going crazy?

Get on any social media site, watch prime time TV, the latest movie, or listen to today's music and you will be bombarded by themes of sex, intimacy, commitment, and betrayal. While being single is portrayed as fun and exciting, the world of coupleship is assumed to be most people's ultimate goal. Yet confusion exists about intimacy and commitment, and sexual betrayal abounds in our culture.

Most couples, whether married or not, have both spoken and unspoken commitments that sex stays within their relationship; and they will communicate and respect each other's personal needs and boundaries. Their expectation is for unconditional love, but they know that relationships have conditions that need to be negotiated openly. Unfortunately, these commitments and expectations are simply a facade in many people's relationships.

Many women are part of a coupleship riddled with deception, lies, and false perception as a result of their partner's compulsive sexual acting out.

Today, in every neighborhood throughout every community, women are being challenged by the addictive nature of their partner's sexual behavior. Perhaps you are a young wife of nineteen who just discovered that your husband was with another woman within days of your wedding. You feel overwhelmed, realizing you don't know your husband at all. Your parents tried to talk you out of the marriage, and now you are thinking maybe they were right.

You may be the mother of two young children and your husband has just lost his job because he was engaging in internet sex during work hours. Suddenly, you start to put together what you thought was odd behavior with the fact that he has also been doing that at home.

You could be a thirty-eight-year-old mother of two with only a high school education and no work experience, who previously refused to believe rumors about your husband's affairs, but now he's been caught in a federal pornography sting and it's all over the front page of the newspaper.

You could be a stay-at-home mom going crazy with suspicions when your husband travels extensively in his work. You know you've heard a woman's voice in the background in his hotel room when you've called him. He says it's just room service. For several months someone has been calling your home and hanging up when you answer. When you question him, he appeals to your insecurity and your past trust issues with your ex-husband.

Or maybe you're forty-seven years of age, you've masked your shame and confusion about your husband's chronic pornographic activity, and now you are horrified because your children are going to find out about their father's voyeurism. You thought he had stopped that behavior, but the police caught him and this time it looks like it will become public.

Or you could be a sixty-five-year-old grandmother of four who's known for forty-five years that your husband has had one affair after the other. There's nothing particularly different about the current affair that you just discovered; it's just the straw that breaks the camel's back. You leave the relationship.

The truth is you could be any woman. You may have children; you may not. You may have the financial resources to be independent but you stay in the relationship; you may want out but your choices are limited because you're financially dependent on your partner. You could be of any faith. In some cases your faith may offer direction and comfort, or you may feel trapped as a consequence of the constrictions of your religion. Your ethnicity and culture may help you stay in denial and normalize behavior that you find hurtful and shaming. Then again, your culture may be what offers you strength and support at a time of great confusion. Perhaps finding yourself in this situation is a family tradition. Generations of women in your family have denied, tolerated, and rationalized the sexual acting out of their men.

No matter who you are or what your background is, to be in a relationship with someone you love, someone you believe loves you, someone you have a commitment with, only to realize he has been acting out sexually is one of the greatest betrayals.

What I want you to know is that you are not alone. There is a path out of this painful situation. From my forty years of professional experience in the addiction and behavioral healthcare field, I am convinced you will find healing happens when you allow yourself the benefit of getting to know others who have walked this path before you and who will now walk alongside you. As you read *Deceived* you'll hear the voices of some brave women who found the courage to confront their truth, to stop living their life in reaction to someone else's behavior, and to trust that they deserve better. These women courageously stepped out of the secrecy to seek direction and, with that, hope. They represent what is only a handful of people—at this time mostly women, but periodically a male in their midst—who found the courage and then the resources to seek out others with whom they could identify. In self-help and therapeutic support groups they found validation for their experiences, they found the support to discover their voices and speak their truths, and they allowed themselves to believe in their worth. Able to let go of their shame and their pain, these women embraced their own strengths within a community of other women who had taken similar paths and most often had similar histories. They would name their community "Women of the Lodge."

Community can mean many things, but for these women it meant a place of belonging and connection. They found other women with whom they could identify—other women who offered an empathetic acceptance of their emotional fragility. As with any community, there were a variety of people and problems, but there was a coming together at a time of crisis for support and in recovery for mutual celebration. As they individually and collectively moved through uncharted emotional and relational territory, they became each other's safety net. The phrase "Women of the Lodge" meant different things to the different personalities, but "Lodge" implied they had come together to be with each other in a place that offered safety through structure, where they would feel warmth as if it emanated from a fire. In this safe place, they became empowered to find their strengths. They found laughter, joy, hope, connection, and a direction to their lives that fostered their well-being. Their journey to health and wellness began.

You may not know where your community is. Your anger, pain, and shame may be so great that you don't even believe you want a community. But it is my belief that by picking up this book, you too are a brave soul who wants validation, support, direction, and hope. This is the beginning of community. You can embark on your journey to health and wellness.

Meet the Women of the Lodge

THERESE

Five years into our marriage I discovered my husband had been regularly viewing pornography and engaged in sex chat rooms on the net. I didn't understand why he would do that because I always tried to please him in bed. I remember crying and telling him it wasn't right. Why wasn't I enough? I really tried to shame him about it, and am sure I did, but he just got better at hiding his behavior. I'd periodically find out that he was still viewing pornography by seeing an email or finding a hidden file on the computer. Each time I'd get "holier than thou" and scold him like I was a punitive mother. I'd call him a hypocrite in the eyes of the Lord, use the bad parent guilt trip, and then off we'd go to church as the perfect family.

I ran our house with an iron fist and always had a smile on my face for the world to see. My children are beautiful and we always went everywhere as the perfect family. My husband had all the criteria for my family picture. He was fun, good-looking, attended church, and never confronted me.

I also became a source of endless questions. I incessantly asked him whether or not he had been on the internet, if he found my women friends attractive, what it was that made them attractive, and if I was prettier than his female coworkers. These questions were intended to make me feel as if I was the only one he'd ever want to be with sexually, somehow believing he had no need for anyone else. I would use my sexuality as a tease, but I really controlled our sex life and often used the kids and illness as an excuse to avoid sex.

Then right about the time I would get comfortable that he was not into pornography anymore, he would be back at it. The next thing I knew, I had an affair—only one, but I felt so self-righteous. I just didn't understand why he did these things. I became really angry and my way of getting back at him was to spend money. I would go on shopping binges and wait for him to say something to me. He never did. I knew he wouldn't. And I knew why.

I loved my husband and I wanted my marriage. A lot of our life was good, but we had this secret life. His lies, his deception, his pornography. My acts of revenge, my shame, my lies to myself and the world. Our screaming at each other, or rather my forever rants full of questions and his passive puppy-dog-look response.

Ultimately, through our church, we found some help with people who knew about sex addiction.

That took away a lot of the shame. I thought that life would be better now. But I stayed totally preoccupied with what he was doing . . . was he going to the therapy groups he said he was going to? Did he connect with women there? Does he have a secret computer somewhere outside of the home? I was busy with the kids at school, but was now isolating from the other moms thinking that maybe they were the ones he chatted with on the internet. I found myself getting angry with the kids for no good reason. It was as if once he started to get better, I felt even more out of control.

As Therese was first learning about her husband's behavior she did what a lot of women do in their shame, in their attempt to deny their humiliation and embarrassment, she moved into Perfectionism. She did what she could to paint a different picture than the reality of what she was living. As long as she stayed busy being the mother to her four children, with a smile on her face, she somehow felt she had control of her world. Just "slice half of me off" is how she referred to what she was doing to cope. She was seeking control where she could, trying to bring some semblance of safety into her life. She was also incredibly enraged, finding ways to both punish her husband and to induce guilt to get him to stop his acting out.

Some women claim emphatically that they would accept internet sex any day over other behaviors. Yet when the behavior is addictive, women whose husbands are engaged in non-physical sex addiction such as pornography, voyeurism, and exhibitionism say they feel the betrayal, the humiliation, and the shame as do those whose partners are engaged in sexual behavior that has become physically intimate with others.

✸ ✸ ✸

Use of the internet to access pornography and/or engage in a virtual sex encounter known as *cybersex* is escalating at alarming rates. Cybersex is much more graphic and hard-core than the porn of magazines many years ago. Things that many people never dreamed sexually are depicted with such detail that nothing is left to the imagination. The neurochemical release is more quickly addicting to the viewer. It results in brain chemistry changes very similar to the high that comes from using certain illegal drugs. Today's internet porn is also more likely leading into chat room experiences, virtual sex, and physical contact with others outside of the computer.

As a consequence of cybersex in particular we are seeing overwhelming escalation in the numbers of marriages being impacted.

Viewing pornography has been associated with a decrease in interest in relationship sexual intimacy. There is an increase in egocentric sexual practices aimed at personal pleasure and with little regard to the pleasure of the engaging partner. There is an increase in the belief that sexual satisfaction can be obtained without affection or emotional attachment; an increase in the belief that relationships are sexually confining; greater dissatisfaction with their partner's physical appearance, sexual performance, and sexual curiosity; and a greater number of requests for sexual practices that partners find objectionable or demeaning. So yes, compulsive engagement in pornography, which is now predominantly cybersex is both hurtful to coupleships and traumatizing to the partner.

Some view pornography as a normal part of adolescence and adulthood while others cast moral judgment on it. Regardless of bias, what you need to remember is that we are talking about the compulsivity of these behaviors. You may be enraged and scared. Like any compulsive behavior, compulsive masturbation and engagement in cybersex warrant attention.

C. S. Lewis writes of the man who masturbates (without engaging directly with another person) as having a harem of imaginary brides. And this harem works against his ever getting out and really uniting with a real human. Think of the tremendous advantages of the harem. It is always accessible, always subservient, calls for no sacrifices or adjustments, and can be endowed with erotic and psychological attractions, which no real person can rival. "Among those shadowy brides he is: always adored, always the perfect lover, no demand is made on his unselfishness, no mortification ever imposed on his vanity. In the end, they become merely the medium through which he increasingly adores himself."[1]

VANESSA

I met my husband at work. He was ideal for me. Charming, smart, but most important to me, he adored me, put me on a pedestal, and needed me. He and I made a great team. He was a loner with low self-esteem and I was the face of confidence, popular, top of the class, and going places. He was broken and looking to be rescued, and I was always looking for a project to save. He excelled under my tutelage and became more successful than he had ever imagined. We were both thrilled with our results. Sadly, this is no foundation for a relationship and I believe he felt like a fraud and coped, as he always had, by sexually acting out. I took his professional accomplishments as another boost to my esteem and became even more grandiose. My career was rocketing, my husband project was doing well, and all was good in my fairy-tale world. I had a perfect life.

I lived in the fast lane—working and partying. My work addiction was modeled on my parents, and I was relentless with the time and energy I poured into getting to the top. What I did not know, with so much time and effort expended on my interests and active party scene, was that my husband, who proclaimed to be ever swamped with work and still a loner, was very busy with other things—namely, other women. For our entire relationship he had been medicating his own feelings of inadequacy, believing he was not good enough, by acting out sexually in every way imaginable. Compulsive daily masturbation, cybersex, internet affairs, and infidelity that ranged from one-night stands to longstanding affairs, from unknowns he picked up over the internet to women he worked with, regular women in multiple cities he traveled to on business, prostitutes, and escorts. Risky sex, unprotected sex in public places, sex in our home, bisexual encounters, and sex with other couples. It was constant and progressive.

All of this was happening and I was happily oblivious, partly because denial was such a learned coping mechanism for me from my growing-up years, and partly because I was so caught up in my own addictions of work and crazy living. As a child

I was very quick to figure things out and with my straight-A marks, compliant demeanor, and affable personality, I excelled in school. I excelled at most anything I put my mind to. So I naturally assumed I was excelling at this marriage. What was it that drove me so hard? The need to prove I was okay, the strong desire for acceptance and approval, the inherent core belief that I wasn't good enough? The truth was that my family was foundationally broken. I was raised by parents in a loveless, work-addicted marriage and subjected to controlling silence and terrifying rages.

From a young age, I was set up to believe that I wasn't of value; therefore, I was meant to be abused by men. This played out for years with the duality of my life: a seemingly perfect persona on the outside and brokenness on the inside, ever driven by my core belief of not being good enough.

But today I realize I had chosen a mate who was also a master deceiver. As smart as I was, he was smarter when it came to deception. So here we were in our dance, me running as fast as I could, living this fun, exciting life, oblivious to the reality of a very fractured coupleship. Then one day before the birth of my son, I was told I had a sexually transmitted disease (STD) that threatened my health and the health of our unborn baby. That was the beginning of my husband telling me about some of his behavior. I was devastated, shocked, overwhelmed, and pregnant. Fortunately, I was able to have a caesarean and the baby was born healthy, and I was treated as well.

Having a child though would create shifts for both my husband and me. We both knew we couldn't go on like this forever and our lives needed to change. But it was really just the beginning, he told me some of his past, and little of his present. I would catch him in lies, I had become the master detective. I was not going to be duped again.

Vanessa, whom you just met, and Jacque, whom you are about to meet, are professional women in their thirties. They take great pride in their work accomplishments; work is a primary source of their esteem. Busyness is a common defense that helps women stay in denial. Slowing down would give them time to analyze their feelings and to ponder the nuances of their partner's behavior that are niggling at their consciousness.

Vanessa's work addiction, her partying, and her image of the good life override her ability to recognize that she is in a relationship with someone who is already engaged in compulsive sexual behavior. Consequently, she is shocked at the unmistakable realization that her husband has a problem. For Jacque, the signs that something was not okay sexually were blatant on the first date, but she readily doubts herself and gives her partner the benefit of the doubt. Jacque more clearly represents the woman who on some level is aware immediately, has profound moments of shame and fear, but works diligently to ignore them. What both of these women recognize in hindsight is how their original family dynamics influenced their frequently unhealthy coping skills. Partners of sex addicts are often raised in addictive, abusive, or otherwise impaired family systems.

JACQUE

"Turn on the TV," a commanding voice in my head said. I didn't usually listen to myself, and I wasn't often home to watch daytime talk shows. I always thought people who sat watching that drivel were pathetic, but the voice persisted so I reached over the sofa on my way out of the room to grab the remote and clicked on the TV. My premonition of drivel and pathetic people was immediately confirmed by the whining I heard from the woman describing her husband's affairs, viewing of pornography, and various other tawdry lowlife events. I didn't need to watch this crap. Yet my feet were cemented to the floor and my fingers refused to click the off button on the remote. I found myself leaning on the couch to listen and pretty soon I hopped over the back and made myself comfy, while with unbelieving ears I listened to several couples describe their walk with sex addiction. "Whew," the louder but unsteady voice in my head said, "Thank God this isn't my problem." Yet a quieter, steadier, and stronger voice kept repeating, "This *is* my life." I clicked the show off as it ended, hopped up, and kept hearing the voice that said, "This *is* my life." And in my ever-present inability to listen to myself, I walked out of the room saying to myself, ". . . and there is nothing I can do about it."

I had been married for just over eleven years and had accomplished much in my career—accolades and awards galore. Yet I felt no joy. I only felt empty, alone, numb, and afraid. I didn't listen to myself. I looked outside of me to the things I did and the reactions of people around me to know how I was doing and feeling. As a matter of fact, if you had asked me to describe how I felt, I would have told you that life was good; I had a great marriage and an awesome family; and I had a wonderful childhood, and let me fix you too!

During this time, my husband was working several miles away and was often gone three to five nights per week. We rarely talked on the phone, and when we did talk, it was superficial. We'd talk about the house and the dogs, and I can remember him telling me that he was attending events with a colleague from work. "She's just a friend," he would tell me. I convinced myself this was normal. In time I would come to find out that she was not his first affair.

When we were together, our only connection was through sex that was always initiated by my husband. It felt mechanical. It was all about arousal and strength and number of orgasms. I agreed to, participated in, and endured this to keep him from getting angry. I convinced myself that our sexual life was normal and healthy. Buried in the tornado of thoughts, an occasional thought that something was wrong would rise to the surface and just as quickly, like a leaf floating in a whirlpool, it would be sucked back down into the depths of my brain.

Prior to meeting my husband, I had several serious boyfriends. I had ended the relationship with my first serious boyfriend (the one everyone assumed I would marry) because he started drinking more than I was comfortable with. My father is an alcoholic, and at age nineteen I had already made a decision that I would not marry an alcoholic. I even made a point to look for someone who didn't drink much and who had a sense of responsibility around alcohol.

I met my husband one year after I completed college. He seemed nice enough and funny, but at the time I had decided I was not dating for a while because of several hurtful encounters. But one day, in a moment of weakness, I agreed to have dinner with him. After dinner, despite my request to go home, he took me to his house. To make a long story short, I liked him, he asked me to stay the night; I said yes but told him we would not be having sex, and he said that was fine with him. I trusted that this would be what happened. And of course I ignored myself when in the middle of the night he initiated sex. I gave in and started a pattern in our relationship that continued for several years. For years I have acquiesced to his requests and ignored my needs, wants, and desires. I did this for the sake of keeping peace.

One of the things that attracted me to my husband was his creativity and knowledge about sex. At first it was exciting to be with someone who seemed to know so much and who suggested so many fun and different things to do sexually. But as our relationship continued to evolve, the fun and creative sex started to become more daring, more outrageous, and more frightening to me.

I started to refuse. He would beg, cajole, and then get angry and I would give in. During sex he would want me to talk dirty to him or look at pornography or fantasize about sex with my female friends and later with male friends. The more I refused, the more he seemed to demand it. He said he had needs and a good wife should meet them. I would feel bad and give in.

Early in our marriage he purchased pornographic stories so we could read them together. He took me to a nude beach; it seemed thrilling but also disgusting. I felt very uncomfortable, and again I chalked it up to me not being as worldly about sex as he was. I found myself drinking to lose inhibitions to do sexual things to please my husband. During this time, my husband started to engage in chat rooms on the internet. When I demanded he stop (because it was too expensive), he told me he wouldn't need to do these things if I would meet his needs and do the things he asked. I felt guilty and degraded. I believed I was worthless for not meeting his needs, but at the same time it seemed wrong. During our marriage, I often suspected things weren't normal. I had such fear of speaking my piece and displeasing my husband. After all, I grew up in a home where my dad raged, yelled, kicked the dog, slammed doors, and threatened violence when he was displeased. Having often feared for my life due to sexual abuse by an older brother, I was easily shamed by men who were intimidating.

My friends frequently told me that my husband made sexualized comments to them. I shrugged it off and buried my feelings regarding any upset I had. History had proven that if I did say something or if I questioned him, he would call me a prude and get angry. He often suggested I was the one with the problem because of my childhood history of sex abuse.

Time passed and it was more of the same, with the chat room time escalating. We were moving around some. I thought changing where we lived would solve everything. What a fantasy. In time, there were more job problems. Well that is what I called them. There were job problems because he was sexually harassing coworkers. Then there were money problems. About this time, his employer suggested we attend a workshop to figure out our lives so I signed us up to go. At this weekend workshop, we admitted to each other that we had both had an affair; we opened up, cleared our consciences, and apologized. I thought we were cured. We continued to attend the workshops and our lives seemed to be improving.

One morning during our common ritual—he insisting on sex, me saying no, he telling me I don't meet his needs—he suddenly blurted out he was having another affair. I just cringed and screamed, "How could you? How could you tell me this while I am on my way to work?" He seemed contrite and remorseful. He apologized and said he thought he might be a sex addict. I remember telling him, "Yeah, right. Sounds like a great excuse." I went to work and we never talked of it again, at least not for a few years.

Over the next couple of years, when I saw flirtatious behavior, I simply ignored it. Then one night when we were in Las Vegas my husband asked me to join him at a sex club. I refused. He insisted, and then he belittled, berated, and cajoled me. I finally gave in. I knew it was wrong, yet I could not say no. I didn't know how to say no and mean it. I was afraid of losing my marriage. I had made up my mind that when I got married, I was married for life. I thought I was stuck with nowhere else to go. I was afraid. I thought I couldn't support myself, despite the fact I had an awesome job with great benefits. I gave in and went to the sex club. There were many people there, some watching, some having sex. I was pressured into performing oral sex. Initially

I refused, but as usual I wasn't strong enough to stand firm or walk away. I felt degraded and dirty. When we got back to the hotel he insisted on having sex. I was worn down, unable to say no anymore, and had sex just to get him to leave me alone. So here we were in full-blown sex addiction and, believe it or not, at the same time taking life-improvement workshops.

I was so afraid of being alone, so afraid of financial instability. Yet I was so alone. I felt like I was sitting at the bottom of a well, the walls slippery and slimy with no way out. I began to cry and it was as if I couldn't stop. My husband told me that he was leaving me for another woman. During a phone session with the life coach, I shared my story with her. And this is how the chapter of recovery started. I began my work, and I don't know why, but when I told my husband what I believed to be true, that he is a sex addict, he began his work as well.

While the addict is frequently engaged in compulsive behavior at the time he marries or forms a coupleship, his partner is often an object in his acting out. Jacque repeatedly engaged in sexual behaviors that denigrated her. Her low self-esteem and fears of abandonment set her up to rationalize her behavior and to be a participant. Jacque was also intimidated, cajoled, manipulated, and controlled by her partner's anger and rage. This is common during life with a sex addict. All of this was strongly fueled by the shame-based beliefs Jacque internalized about herself and is similar to Vanessa's lack of belief in her own worth and value.

SARA

Twenty-four years ago, after two divorces, I married the man I thought was absolutely the most wonderful, successful, and admirable man one could hope for. He had me with his first hello. Looking back, I know today there were signs that Mr. Wonderful might have some problems: he gawked at attractive and sleazy-looking women; he drank to drunkenness on more than a few occasions; he went into rages when something didn't go the way he wished; and he had a sort of disconnectedness during sex. I was concerned enough prior to getting married that I went to a therapist and confronted my then fiancé about my fears. I was quickly told by both my husband and the therapist that I was projecting the behaviors I had experienced with my two previous husbands onto my fiancé, a very successful and upstanding man.

Having a history of being willing to trust others rather than myself, I unquestioningly went on with the wedding. On our honeymoon, my husband shared some of his sexual past that he had not previously shared. My heart went cold as he described encounters with prostitutes, friends, relatives, and so on. Knowing what I know now, I see it as a classic description of sex addiction. I was horrified, terrified, and literally frozen with the sinking feeling that I had married someone weird. I freaked out.

We limped through our honeymoon and I made up my mind to put all his past behind us and forge ahead with a positive effort to make a good home for my three children, ages ten through sixteen. The years added up, filled with my husband's rages, drinking, flirting, and ogling women with abandon. We had countless arguments about his behavior and he would point to my theatrical behavior as just crazy. He was right: I was feeling crazy. I was terrified that I had made another bad marriage, that I was not desired, that I couldn't explain how hurt I was, and that he would never change.

We both spent countless hours in therapy, together and individually. The children had problems, and life was never easy or peaceful. After a crisis with one of our kids, my husband confessed to me that he had been unfaithful on several occasions. He was fired from each executive position he had. I had to leave graduate school and go back to work for financial reasons. My desperation grew and grew until I thought I must be clinically crazy. I was constantly threatening him. My anger and resentment built up to the point where I told myself, "Hell, if you can't beat them, then just join them!" I had a short revenge affair with my boss but quickly realized that was not what I wanted or who I was. It didn't help my hurt or anger. In fact it made my misery even worse, having dented my self-respect.

One night after I had been diagnosed with early stage breast cancer, I discovered a book about sex addiction in the trunk of the car. When I questioned him, my husband said his therapist wanted him to read it, as he thought my husband was a sex addict. Well, I took the book straight into the living room of our house, sat down, and flew through every page. My first reaction was "Oh my God, I am not crazy after all. This is our life!" What followed was his agreement that this seemed to be what, in fact, we were living with. He confessed to having had sex with several massage prostitutes. I calmly told him we were finished. Before when he had confessed to affairs, I had told him if he ever did it again, we were through.

We separated. In time, we began to talk about moving back together, and I told him for us to get back together he had to go to a treatment program. He agreed. By now in between radiation treatments I was working with a therapist. She had me looking at my reactivity, fears, resentments, and my attempts at controlling the insane world around me. Here I had kids at home, cancer, a husband I couldn't trust, and my own past trauma. The funny part to me was that my therapist kept telling me to "take a deep breath."

A few years back my husband quit drinking and began attending Alcoholics Anonymous (AA) meetings. He kept going to meetings right through this sexual acting out, and our separation, etc. I have now been in Al-Anon for the past five years. As crazy as I felt, the teachings of Al-Anon were helpful; it was just that I didn't know most of the time what I was even living with.

Because of her experience with Al-Anon, Sara is a woman with a solid understanding of addiction, which makes it easier for her to accept her husband's sexual acting out as an addiction. But while she is living in the throes of deceit, not wanting another failed marriage, trying to raise kids, she finds herself in a state of reaction versus action. With the acknowledgment of her husband's behavior being sex addiction, she draws on her Al-Anon experience and feels hope as she believes in the process of recovery that comes with honesty. Yet, she also knows she needs more than Al-Anon to help her address the impact of ongoing sexual betrayal. With that history, she moves forward with her life.

Through the ensuing months, there spilled out the rest of the confessions about money spent on one of my husband's victims, friends he had sex with, other sordid details that I had frankly conveniently forgotten. But I do remember the pain of how we struggled. I ranted. I got angrier and angrier. I can remember early in my husband's recovery when he was becoming honest with me and I thought, *I don't know that I can stand the pain.* Between the breast cancer and the hurt of my husband's sexual acting out, it felt like I was sinking into a big black hole. It was at this time my therapist saved my life by saying, "You can either get revenge by continuing to yell and threaten; or get a divorce and feel better temporarily; or you can roll up your sleeves, get to work on yourself, and feel better for the rest of your life." That simple piece of advice has given me my life back. The work has been painful, exhausting, and sometimes embarrassing, but I have me, I have a life of which I am proud, and I have the integrity I always wanted.

We went to conferences, therapy, recovery meetings, therapeutic weekends, and on and on. I expected absolute immediate recovery on both our parts. That did not happen. But what did happen was that I found me. I began to live what I have always wanted: an honest life. We were separated for nearly a year, and during this time I realized that since we had lived so long in the disease and we were both actively pursuing recovery, we might try doing that together. It has not all been uphill; it has been more like a roller coaster. I lapse into hypervigilance when feeling insecure, and we struggle yet with our sex life. In general we both want our marriage to be better, and we work on it both individually and together.

As you have just read, after two divorces Sara thought she had met Mr. Wonderful, her soul mate. He was charming, fun, good-looking, and a great provider, and he embraced her children. With the information her husband shared with her on their honeymoon, she didn't know how to cope with what she perceived would be another failed relationship. Wanting to trust herself, she sought out counseling but was frequently told to give her husband the benefit of the doubt. During much of their marriage, her insides were screaming at the subtle and the blatant behaviors. As she says, "The worms were moving." As is typical with trauma victims, her intuition was trying to claim its voice, but fear and shame often overshadowed it. Sara frequently appeared more out of control in her rage than her husband did in his acting out. Challenged with raising children who were struggling, and with learning the full truth about his behavior, she was also faced with a serious health problem. In my work with women, I have found that as they confront the issues of their fractured relationships, they are still faced with multiple challenges of life, such as caretaking of sick parents, losing their parents, parenting children, or health concerns of their own or their partners. People don't get to choose the time to have major life issues present themselves.

MAITE

Twenty years ago, as a young adult, I came to the United States from South America. In my culture, it is perceived as normal and generally accepted that men will have mistresses and affairs. The men think those affairs make them look richer and more masculine. Women are never to complain, especially in public. In some way, as the wife, you are the honored one, the chosen one. You are the Madonna, the one he loves because he married you. That is supposed to be enough for any woman. But I wanted something different. Knowing that I was coming to America, and that in America women had voices and power and men had less pressure to be macho, I had my big wedding and got married. I thought my marriage would be perfect; there would be no infidelity. Three days after my wedding, my husband told me that he had gotten another woman pregnant and she was having the baby.

Surprise, surprise—my marriage was a play of pretending, lots of lies and infidelities, lots of deceiving. Here I was in a new country. I didn't know anyone except his family. I didn't speak the language. We were living in his parents' house because our apartment was not ready yet. The worst part was I had no one to talk to.

While growing up I learned I had to be perfect. That was the expectation from friends and family members. My father and mother were community leaders, very involved in politics, church, and education. I saw my father as a perfect dad, and he had high dreams of me helping humanity. My mother was the perfect educator and received multiple awards. There was a whole community watching and raising me. We were never to disagree; we were to believe and feel the way our parents or the church said or did. I was the most perfect child, accelerating through school, graduating high school as class valedictorian (of course), and rapidly moving through Catholic law school. Then to the surprise of my parents, I got married immediately after graduation.

My marriage would not be blessed as I had willed it to be. Over the years I would find out about things that were going on. Women would call my house and tell me things about my husband. Or someone at his work would pull me aside and tell me to open my eyes. There were hundreds of women. I would try to find out what I could before I would accuse him, and then I would be so self-righteous. I would find credit card slips from restaurants and hotels where he had no reason to be. I found receipts for women's presents that I did not receive. He bought perfume I did not wear. He had dinner vouchers for more than one other person. I became quite the investigator, quite the interrogator. I would check his luggage and plane tickets; a lot of his acting out took place when he was away from home on work-related trips. I would not talk to him for days; I would not sleep with him. When I would confront him I would give him an ultimatum. I would tell him, "I can have a better life. I am going back home." He would freeze; he would say nothing. I would move out of our bedroom for a few weeks, and then in time he would say he was sorry and act like he was ashamed. He would beg me to give him another chance. And time after time I would.

The worst part is that much of the time I knew the women he was seeing. Ninety-nine percent were women who knew me. I knew them in my committee work, my fundraising work, or they were friends. I did not ever say anything to them.

Within just a few years of my marriage I was seriously looking for answers as to what was wrong. I prayed for help in seeing the light.

I began to read books about women and oppression. I was looking at how class and gender impact women and men differently. I was reading about the role of money and how the more money a man has, the greater imbalance of the relationship in the marriage. I was reading that money was power, and the more power, the greater the abuse in marriages. I was beginning to see myself as a feminist and trying to understand my life from a feminist perspective. In that process, I began to see how he would use these women and then dispose of them like tissue paper. Then I began to see this was not about having an affair, this was something much bigger; something much sicker, worse than I could ever imagine. By now I was living my worst nightmare, and I was alone, disconnected, and powerless. I was angry at God, and in all of that I was pretending things were better and happier than they were.

When we got married I was a size two. I knew I was attractive, so why did he want someone else? Then as I got older, and after I had kids, I started to gain weight, and when I was in my mid-thirties, my body began to change. He would tell me he needed a younger woman. I knew he was with younger women then. I would do things like bleach my hair, exercise a lot, and go to the beauty parlor all of the time. I would dress sexy. I would do all of these things and nothing I did made a difference. This just made it worse for me, trying to please someone who I couldn't please.

Over the years, I went to as many as fifteen therapists. Sometimes I would get my husband to go. We were in therapy within the first two weeks of our marriage. But I was always seen as the one who simply wasn't happy here in the United States. I was told we had communication problems. Well, maybe my English was not so great, but my Spanish was just fine. I continued to ask for help, but I didn't get the help I needed.

His addiction was progressing. He was becoming more secretive with his behavior and hiding it within his workplace. There was eventually the threat of a lawsuit because it appeared he had nonconsensual sex with a coworker.

But let me remind you, I was still working very hard to be the perfect wife. We tried to keep our arguing very private so the kids did not see. But the kids were now teenagers and they would ask, "How can we be the perfect family when Daddy has two other kids and Mommy is not the mother?"

Then not too many years ago, my mother told me about my father's infidelities. I thought my father was very religious and would never do that. I felt so dumb because all of these years I thought I had perfect parents, and then I married someone who has affairs. I thought I should have known better. I beat myself up. So when my mother told me this, I understood that I was not dumb. This is a part of my family history and I am repeating that history. Throughout my family, other women were a part of the men's lives.

Finally I told my husband I had had enough. I was leaving; I could not stand the emptiness in me; and I could no longer keep pretending and faking. Everyone thought we had this fairy-tale marriage, that we were the perfect couple. I knew it was not that way and never had been. I knew I loved him, but because I love myself as well, I had to leave. I hadn't been true to myself for too many years. I was a beautiful package but there was nothing inside. I knew we loved each other, but something bigger was destroying our relationship.

I remember telling my children that I was not happy with their father and that I needed to breathe. I told them I needed to find out what was wrong with me. I blamed myself. My husband said he didn't know what was wrong with me either. We have separated and I know I need to focus on me. I am totally distraught and totally obsessed with him still. My weight is a roller coaster overmedicating with food and then trying to look like the women I imagine him with. But I am going to take care of me and hopefully change things for my children.

Maite presents a picture of how culture can support a man's sexual acting out and how that consequently makes it more difficult for her to trust and honor herself. This was a marriage where she knew early on about his affairs and even about his other children. Regardless of culture, it is not uncommon for a child to be born as a consequence of the acting-out behavior. Maite became aware of these other children when they were still babies, whereas in many situations the female partner may not find out for years. Many times the father secretly supports the child and is even involved in the parenting.

As is true of many partners, Maite repeatedly sought professional help. Unfortunately, like others, she was often told that she was overreacting and bore unwarranted suspicions. When Maite talks about acting crazy, she is referring to being in a full-blown trauma response. Her behavior is much more the norm, it is not about being crazy.

In this final story, Jenny also realizes early on that her husband is sexual with other women. She trusts her own intuition but feels emotionally and financially trapped; she wants to try to make her marriage work. She quickly learns that to be able to stay without going crazy, she has to accept his rationalizations, thereby losing her sense of true self, another response to the trauma of betrayal.

JENNY

The first time I found out my husband had been unfaithful I was eighteen years old, four months pregnant, and seven months into a marriage that I didn't really want to be in. So eighteen, married, pregnant, and deciding to give it my all, deciding to love him, believe in him, trust him, he comes home one night and I knew immediately that something was different with him. He was closed off a little, he was good at acting normal but I could sense the slightest change in him. I didn't push the issue until later that night when I just kept asking him what had gone on at work that day.

Finally, unable to persuade me that everything was fine, he started to tell me how much he loved me and how he was in love with me and that being in love with me was the most important thing, and that what he did at work didn't have any effect on that. As I listened it was like he was brainwashing me. Then he told me he had had sex with a coworker and how it was okay because she really wanted to do it for him; that it had nothing to do with love and that he loved me and it was just what men need now and then. He continued to drone on like a hypnotist, continuing to try to convince me that it was okay, that I should just accept it and know that it was just sex; that he loved me and that is what mattered; that I knew what he was like before I married him; and that I should just not let it bother me.

I remember taking our wedding picture down off the wall and falling to my knees and crying uncontrollably, grieving the loss of the perfect marriage that I had envisioned; a marriage that I let him talk me into and a pregnancy that I wasn't ready for. I was still a child with a childlike mentality, and he, being fourteen years older, had always been a father figure to me. I trusted him to be faithful and trustworthy. My fantasy was shattered.

In my childlike state, I had no ability to even conceive of leaving the marriage or telling him never to do this to me again; I didn't have the emotional resources to be able to do that. So my only psychological option was to believe him. To accept his reality, not mine. It was okay, he loved me; this is what men do. I had to believe a bunch of lies and make them my own in order to survive the situation that I found myself in. It was the only way I could psychologically survive. I told myself that he wouldn't do this again, especially because he saw how much it hurt me, and I knew he didn't want to hurt me because he said he loved me. So I rationalized that my brokenness and pain would stop him from ever being unfaithful to me again. He just kept minimizing it and telling me that I was overreacting, that I didn't realize that this is what all men do and that I shouldn't be so upset by this. It really was no big deal, it was just sex! I guess the insinuation was that sex had nothing to do with love and that he loved me. As a very young woman, I found it mind-twisting.

For twenty more years, Jenny went in and out of acknowledging that her husband's addictive behavior was abusive. She was a master of her own deception. She frequently felt she had to engage in his sexual fantasies, even telling herself it was okay. Her life was on autopilot. She continued to relate to her husband as if she was the child, although she tapped into adult strengths in her parenting skills. She saw no way out of the situation, and that path did not show itself for a number of years. In many ways, Jenny was like a hostage bonded to a captor—the Stockholm syndrome. The dynamics that lead to such extreme bonding are 1) the presence of a perceived threat to one's physical or psychological survival and the belief the abuser would carry out out the threat; 2) presence of a perceived small kindness from the abuser; 3) isolation from perspectives of others than those of the abuser; and 4) the perceived inability to escape the situation. While the majority of women involved with men who act out sexually are not experiencing Stockholm Syndrome, many will identify with an attachment and loyalty that is symptomatic of such bonding and defies their own well-being.

Jenny continues to share her journey:

My husband was acting out on all his addictions. Early on I began to live a life of cover-up and compensation. And I became busier and busier and more and more distant from him. I was seriously trauma bonded with my husband. There was a complete loss of self into the other. I had no idea of the trauma that I allowed myself to be subjected to by accepting my husband's infidelity and his excuses; I rationalized that the pornography was nothing because there was just so much sexuality spewing all over our relationship; I accepted his emotional and verbal abuse of me and the children; I accepted his emotional abandonment through drug abuse and his traumatizing through his fits of rage.

Physically I worked with frenzy in everything I did. Emotionally and spiritually everything was mechanized. There was no emotional connection. Buried anger and exhaustion eventually sent me into such a depressed state of being that I was unable to function, even at the most minimal level. At that time, about sixteen years into our marriage, I went through two severe depressions and a nervous breakdown. These rendered me completely unable to do anything. My ability to hide behind accomplishment and being capable vanished. I became a mental midget.

Even the simplest task of looking up a phone number would send me into fits of tears. Balancing a checkbook or even writing a check was no longer possible for me. I couldn't think, concentrate, or handle pressure or responsibility of any kind. My husband began to drink heavily, and rages were the norm. I had lost the ability to cope.

It was at this point that I turned to a power greater than myself. I asked Jesus into my heart and told him I couldn't do this alone. That started my spiritual healing. I prayed that Jesus would change my husband, change my circumstances, but it was not until I asked him to change me that things started to change. This is when I began to address the trauma that had permeated this marriage.

Jenny began her journey by reaching out to her faith community and seeking guidance; Therese was directed to a counselor through her church; Vanessa and Jacque began their journeys forward at the height of crisis, Vanessa by contracting an STD during pregnancy, and Jacque when watching her husband walk out the door to be with another woman. Maite's healing began at the time she was prepared to leave her marriage. Sara came across a book that her husband was reading as he began to come to terms with the fact that he had another addiction—sex. Whatever the impetus or crisis is that directs you to begin a healing journey, you have the potential of living your life differently.

Moving On to Your Journey

The deception and betrayal women experience takes many forms. Knowingly or unknowingly, you are touched by it daily. For some, it is pornography or fantasies with faceless names on the internet. For others, it is the other women who may be one-night stands, a coworker, your best friend, escorts, or prostitutes. It may involve voyeurism, exhibitionism, or bisexual behavior. Often other addictions, depression, and rage issues all serve to complicate matters.

The pain for those in a relationship with someone acting out sexually is undeniable. You have been betrayed, deceived, and lied to. Your vows have been violated again and again. You have been ignored or manipulated emotionally and physically. You may have been asked to engage in sexual practices that you found repulsive and abusive. You may realize he has been or is currently in a long-term relationship that involves financial commitments and possibly even children. You may have been placed at risk of contracting sexually transmitted diseases. These offenses lead to a wide range of thoughts and feelings, from despair, anger, hurt, and desperation to wondering and pleading for answers.

To be in a deceptive relationship, whether you are conscious of it or not, frequently results in the following traumatic responses:

- Feeling crazy

- Lying to yourself and to others

- Not trusting yourself

- Having emotional outbursts

- Feeling anguished

- Denying

- Suspicions

- Being emotionally numb

- Walking on eggshells

- Defending yourself with busyness or perfectionism

- Being depressed

- Burying your head in the sand; ignoring signs

- Experiencing health problems

- Changing yourself to please, accommodate, or pacify

- Feeling inadequate

- Being obsessive

- Socially withdrawing

- Having rageful thoughts and behavior

- Acting out via food, alcohol, drugs, spending, or affairs

Chapter Two, In the Face of Truth, will explore more fully the many behaviors and feelings characteristic of being in a relationship impacted by sexual compulsivity. It will also help you to understand more how what is occurring leads not just to attempts to cope but results in traumatic responses.

As painful as the stories are, there is hope. The women you've just met are all joyfully living their lives differently as a consequence of changes they have made. Throughout this book, you will continue to hear from them, as well as many other unnamed partners who give voice to their journey. Like the Women of the Lodge, you, too, have the strength to move forward in your life. Understanding what has happened and recognizing how you are impacted can lead to a life-changing transformation. It takes courage; it is painful. But the possibilities of living your life differently are worth the struggle. My hope is that you will allow yourself to begin this journey.

Reflective Thoughts and Questions

- Underline or highlight the parts of the women's stories with which you identify.

- Which behaviors sound familiar to you?

- Is there any particular woman whose story sounds similar to yours? In what way?

- What feelings did you experience as you read this chapter? Relief? Sadness? Anger? Fear? Hope? Loneliness? Shame? Others?

- What was important for you to learn in this chapter?

CHAPTER ONE NOTES

1   C. S. Lewis, *Collected Letters of C. S. Lewis*, vol. 3 (New York: HarperOne, 2007), 758–59.

CHAPTER TWO

In the Face of Truth

This can't be happening.

What did I do? Is it my fault?

Why do I feel so crazy?

After hearing time after time that you have quite an imagination or that you are the one responsible for his unhappiness or that it's your job to shut up and be grateful for what you have or that you simply have trust issues, you learn to keep quiet. You keep fears and doubts to yourself while your self-esteem erodes away.

[THERESE]

Whenever I confronted my husband with my suspicions that he was interested in other women, he would always say that I was the one he loved. He said that while he found other women interesting to look at, I didn't need to worry. But I did worry. What if he decided to meet someone in one of those chat rooms that I knew about? From there my thinking was all a downhill spin inside my head: I'm not pretty enough, smart enough, or sexy enough.

[PARTNER]

So many times my husband would say, "You are lucky to have me in your life. No other man is willing to take on a woman with four young children. You should just be more grateful and not so controlling all of the time." Then I'd tell myself I have trust issues with men and if I could just be more trusting, everything would really be okay. I try not to act so needy, so desperate, because I think that drives him away, but it is hard for me when I am so scared I will lose him.

[JACQUE]

Well, he basically told me it was about me. He had been telling me I was undersexed. That I just didn't know what a man needed. And I don't seem to enjoy having sex because when we have sex I always end up feeling used or even more alone than when we started. Then I notice other women noticing him, and he them, and I begin to compare myself to them. Maybe they are younger than me or have more money and can dress up better, but no matter—I basically always feel as if I am just not what he wants.

Just as an alcoholic's partner frequently feels guilty for the behavior of the alcoholic—that if he or she was a better partner and could just do the right thing, the alcoholic wouldn't drink so much—partners of men who are acting out sexually nearly always believe that his behavior is a statement about themselves. They believe they must not be pretty enough, sexy enough, smart enough, thin enough, alluring enough, ample-breasted enough, or long-legged enough. The list is never-ending. You are full of "shoulds:" *I should have taken more time for him. I should have been less focused on the kids or work. I should not have let my appearance go. I should have kept my weight down.* Again, it's a never-ending list.

You probably operate from the following belief: I need to do or be something different and that will make him stop. First and foremost you need to understand that you are not the cause of your partner's acting-out behavior. It isn't about you needing to be different. He engages in his activity because of his own emotional wounding, which now manifests in a pathological relationship with a mood-altering behavior—in his case—sex. Chapter Three will help you better understand the addictive nature of his behaviors. But because it's natural when caught in the web of deception to lose focus of self, let's change the dynamic and keep the focus on you.

As lonely as your experience may feel, partners of sex addicts often have much in common with one another, beginning with rationalizing, minimizing, and denying.

Denial: Protecting the Illusion

Living with addiction is poignantly described by a young girl in an addictive family who said, "Denial is when you pretend things are different than how they really are." For years, partners of addicts, regardless of the addiction, have pretended that things are different than how they really are. For both the addict and the partner, denial is at the core of active addiction. When the addictive behavior is sex instead of alcohol or other drugs, gambling, food, and so on, denial for the partner is often accelerated because of the greater degree of shame. While addicts deny in order to satisfy their addiction, partners deny in an attempt to hang on to what is really an illusion, the fantasy that all is really okay. The fact is that life is out of control; the addiction is in the driver's seat. But deny you must when you can't see your way out. It is a form of self-protection.

Denying, minimizing, and rationalizing is a natural response to the insidiousness of addiction. With sex addiction it sounds like:

- "The pornography doesn't really bother me, it's only pictures."

- "If I were more attractive he would not be doing this."

- "He can't help it if other women throw themselves at him."

- "Work must be his problem; if he would just change jobs then things would be different."

- "If we move he will stop this behavior."

Your denial is supported by extensive rationalization. Examples of rationalization include these statements:

- "Men will be men."

- "He is an honest person; he would not lie to me."

- "The lipstick on his collar got there when a coworker asked him to dance. He didn't want to be rude and say no."

- "He's not really staring at women; he's just interested in watching people."

- "He's not flirting, that's just his nature; he's a very friendly guy."

- "We took vows before God. He would not break his vows."

- "He is such a religious man. He takes his faith seriously."

- "It doesn't hurt to look at pictures (porn). At least he is not having an affair."

- "It's easier for him to be friends with women. It doesn't mean he is having an affair."

- "His business calls him away. After all, he does it so the kids and I can have a good lifestyle."

- "His business takes priority over me and the kids, but I understand. It's just while he is building his career."

- "It's important for him to go to business functions without me. I'm not comfortable there, and I have to take care of the kids anyway."

- "I must have gotten this STD from a toilet seat. He told me I couldn't have gotten it from him."

- "Just because they have lunch together doesn't mean they are having an affair. He has to do business with her."

- "He told me the long-distance calls were not his. The phone company must have made a mistake."

- "It's okay if he gives her a Christmas gift; she does work for him."

- "Those internet spammers are infiltrating our email with porn sites."

- "The police are exaggerating his behavior."

- "I bet the babysitter called these telephone sex numbers when she was here."

- "This is the way he grew up."

- "He's such a good dad."

- "It's not his fault that I can't fulfill him sexually."

- "I am the one he comes home to."

Does any of the above sound familiar?

When rationalizations become weak, the tendency to minimize comes next. That only strengthens the denial. Minimizations common to those in relationships with sex addicts include statements like these:

- "It's not that bad."

- "I'm the only one who really understands him."

- "He needs me—now more than ever."

- "It's just a phase."

- "It's not his fault that whore went after him; he didn't have a chance."

- "He's so great in all other areas—it's just this one area."

- "I'm not that interested in sex anyway."

- "It could be worse. At least he is not addicted to (something other than sex, such as alcohol, other drugs, or gambling)."

- "It doesn't matter if I don't know everything he does."

How often have you had these thoughts?

Think about the beliefs and fears that bolster your rationalizations and minimizations. Partners of addicts share common beliefs and fears. Some of them are:

- "I can't live without him."

- "I might end up alone, and if I am alone that proves I am not worthy."

- "No one else will ever love me."

- "I don't deserve better."

- "He's the father of my children, and they need their father."

- "All men are like this."

- "If we separated, I would have to give up some aspects of my lifestyle for lack of money."

- "My family might find out and I'd feel humiliated."

- "The kids might find out and I won't know how to handle it.

- "I might have to give up my home."

- "I've never balanced a checkbook, paid bills, or paid attention to our retirement, and I am not capable."

- "If others found out about his sexual behavior they would think I'm not a good sexual partner, because if I were, he would not stray."

- "If he is a sex addict, then all the good times in the past were a lie."

Does any of the above sound familiar?

At this point in your reading, it's easy to start to berate yourself and feel like a fool. If you are beating yourself up, stop. Of course you want to protect yourself. You want to believe it's not the problem it is. You want to give him the benefit of the doubt. Don't be critical of yourself. The truth is excruciatingly painful. It also taps into your shame and humiliation. The illusion of safety and security is an enticing fantasy. Sadly, in the process you quit trusting yourself and your inner voice. But you have begun the process of honoring yourself. You are doing that now in the act of learning about what has been happening and how to take care of yourself.

[PARTNER]

Whatever happened to me, I was made to feel I deserved it; I caused it. I learned not to make waves. I assumed I had no right to complain. So I just put my head in the sand, and whether or not it was denial or whatever, I just wasn't going to deal with it. In my mind I had to make peace.

Denial doesn't mean not having a clue. It often means dismissing the seriousness of the behavior. You don't know what to believe, so out of fear you simply believe what makes you feel safest. Denial stems from a yearning to believe that all will be fine or that all will return to how it was before this acting-out behavior reared its ugly head. The addict lies to you, and now you lie to yourself. Confused by self-deception, you do not take action and you spend your energy reacting or stamping out fires. Denial is the oxygen feeding the fire.

[PARTNER]

I actually found out because he told me. He thought I was going to find out anyway. He apologized, begged me to forgive him, and pleaded with me not to leave, saying it was just this one time and it wouldn't happen again. He told me he had already told his boss he couldn't go on road trips anymore, that he had to be closer to home. So I thought this time maybe this cloud had a silver lining for us. But after a while I noticed he would get off the computer abruptly when I came in. He was late coming home from work or at a ball game with clients. It wasn't clear, but I just had this feeling. He kept telling me he loved me and we were still having good sex. I made sure of that; I initiated it. I would buy sexy clothing that I knew he liked. I thought that meant something, like I was the only one. He often told me what a good mother I was and I know that meant a lot to him, as his mother left him when he was young. Somehow I thought that was so important to him that he wouldn't do anything more to hurt me. I just wanted to trust him, to believe him. So I ignored and dismissed all of my fears and my inner voice. I trusted him when I should have trusted myself.

[SARA]

Time would pass, months, a few years, and I just wanted to believe his words so I turned the other way and got busy. I dove into my job and the kids. Having a family takes time. I remember telling myself he was there for the kids, at their events. But looking back now, that wasn't true. I often had this strange feeling. It was like this little voice in my head, and then I would tell myself more loudly, "He is a good guy. I am lucky to have him. I don't have any reason to not trust him." By then he had owned up to two affairs. Because he cried and asked for forgiveness, I guess I thought that earned him my trust.

Then he got fired for sexual harassment. He told me it wasn't fair, that the woman had actually harassed him, meaning she seduced him. We were having financial problems and I didn't understand why, and now he had no job; we just sort of let the financial stress and the need for him to get a job become our focus. It would be another year before I would know I was just seeing the tip of the iceberg. I so wanted to believe his lies. When I get honest, I realize how frightened I am to be alone. I equate it to not being loved, being unlovable. It is like this failure of a marriage just confirms all I have ever believed about myself: I don't deserve to be loved.

Denial is meant to be a protective defense. It is a natural response to hurt and loss. The fear of what you think you might need to do if you were confronted with the truth is so immobilizing that it reinforces the need to stay in denial.

After all, what does it mean if you don't stay in denial? Does it mean divorce? More arguing? Disrupting the children's lives? A threat to your lifestyle? You are not desirable? Punishment from the church? While you are busy questioning yourself, the addict stands strong in his denial and rationalization, protecting his stash and continuing his addiction.

Denial induces numbness; it is a lot like frostbite. People who get frostbite are often unaware of the damage that is occurring because they simply cannot feel the burn. Now couple your need for denial with the fact that sex addicts are masters of misdirection. They perform sleight-of-hand tricks that create illusions, distort events, and make crises disappear. They can quickly tap into your vulnerability and charm you or shame you right out of your distrust.

GASLIGHTING: MASTER OF MISDIRECTION
The sex addict is highly skilled at performing sleight of hand tricks that create illusions, distort events, and make crises disappear. He or she can quickly tap into your vulnerability and charm you or shame you right out of your distrust.

[ADDICT]

I told myself that what she doesn't know won't hurt her. I work away from home, I work hard, and no one thanks me for it. I was lonely; I deserved some fun. When she would accuse me, rightfully of my many affairs, I would tell her she had guy friends at work, so why can't I have a friendship with a colleague who happens to be a woman? I took on a lawyer mentality. It was easy for me to line up evidence, like I was trying a case. I had proof that I wasn't doing what in fact I was. I would stick to my guns. She didn't need me to line up a lot of evidence because she didn't want to believe it. I knew she was looking to be talked out of her perceptions. My lies, sprinkled with reassurances, gave her something to hold on to, a little life preserver. I know it sounds sick now, but then I was justifying my own behavior. I wasn't thinking about her, or us. My addiction was in control.

[ADDICT]

I was always on the offensive. Even before I walked into the house, I would start to intimidate her. I would call and quickly begin to ask her if she had gotten certain things done that day that I knew she couldn't have. Then I would act exasperated and without saying it I would let her know how disappointed I was. Other times when we would be out publicly I would start to accuse her of flirting or maybe having an affair. The whole time I had affairs going all the time. If she even began to question me I would turn the conversation to things such as telling her how she reminded me of my ex. I didn't like this part of me, but I didn't like any of me. I was just protecting myself and my stash—the other women.

An addict in recovery is very capable of recognizing and admitting to his manipulations. His manipulations may include being charming, bullying, threatening, and playing the victim. Often a combination of these manipulations is used.

[ADDICT]

My partner never wanted to believe what she suspected or was told by others. I knew that. As much as she was upset, I took advantage of the relief I saw in her when I denied it. And that is what I would do: I denied, denied, and denied. If she pushed, and sometimes she did, I would finally just throw up my arms and ask her in a threatening tone, "What do you want? Do you want to leave? Do you want a divorce?" Mostly I used this angry tone to intimidate her, and she would readily back down. I could go on the defense in a second. She would start accusing me and within seconds I would say, "Why don't you just leave?" And that was always followed by name-calling. Oh, I was also real good at trying to make her think there was something wrong with her to be so mistrusting. I would act like I was this victim of her paranoia, that she was the one who was crazy.

This conduct is beyond hurtful. It's cruel, abusive, and traumatizing. There is also a very specific name for it: *gaslighting*. Gaslighting is a strong form of emotional manipulation used to confuse people into thinking their perceptions are so off base that they are crazy. It's a form of abuse in which false information is presented, questions posed, statements made with the intent of making a victim doubt his or her own memory, perception, and sanity.

This term was coined from the 1939 movie *Gaslight* in which a devious husband, played by Charles Boyer, manipulates and torments his wife, played by Ingrid Bergman, to convince her she is going mad, all in an attempt to acquire her jewelry. He can accomplish this by having her certified as insane and hauled off to a mental institution. To do this he intentionally manipulates the gaslights in their home to intermittently flicker off and on. Every time Bergman reacts to it he denies that any flickering is occurring and tells her she is just seeing things.

When people who are determined to keep their secrets begin to be questioned, they often become experts at pushing your buttons, they know your sensitivities and vulnerabilities and use that knowledge against you for you to back off with your suspicions. This behavior often renders many partners emotionally mute.

The consequences to gaslighting for the victim are wide ranging. These include:

- No longer feeling you can trust yourself

- Being more anxious and less confident than you used to be

- Doubting your own perceptions

- Feeling like everything you do is wrong

- Apologizing often

- Consistently thinking there is something wrong with you but unable to identify it

- Making excuses for your partner's behavior

- Avoiding giving information to trusted family or friends in an attempt to avoid confrontation

- Experiencing a greater sense of isolation

- Never feeling safe

- Profound depression

- Anxiety

Is any of the above familiar?

There are very few partners of sex addicts who cannot identify with having lived with this experience and in many cases repetitively for years.

The trauma has begun. What I mean by this is the insidiousness of the deception is becoming chronic. As the addict becomes more and more caught up in his acting out behavior, his addiction is progressing. Behavior such as gaslighting is used more, fueling your insecurities, your self-doubt, and the sense of craziness that can lead to trauma responses.

TOXIC STRESS LEADING TO TRAUMATIC RESPONSES

Trauma is the result of a shock to the body, mind, or soul. It is the body's and the brain's response to a severe painful experience. It can be caused by any stimulus too powerful or too sudden and unexpected to be assimilated or processed in a normal way. It breaks down your psychological defenses and shatters your sense of security.

Historically, when people have thoughts of trauma they think of situations such as a car accident or their home burning to the ground. You may think of acts of war or terrorism or shootings in your community. You may think of a natural disaster such as floods, hurricanes, fires, and tornadoes that occur throughout the year. Yet the majority of people who experience a trauma are more apt to experience something more chronic, not acute, subtler, not as blatant and much more likely to be within their family. For partners who have lived with sex addiction, the trauma is in the chronicity of betrayal, the lying, and the loss of trust.

Our body is designed to recover after short-lived traumas known as acute traumatic events. But ongoing traumas like intimate sexual deceptions where you are exposed to hurtful events repeatedly and over long periods of time are different. You are much more apt to be living in a chronic state of alarm and hypervigilance from both the emotional violations and looming sense of threat to your sense of security, which alters how your body and brain system operates.

Chronic stress experienced, even when unacknowledged, will leave you with a highly dysregulated nervous system, making it difficult to feel secure in the face of any everyday stressor let alone one that is attacking the safety and sanctity of your coupleship.

On a daily basis, our nervous system experiences periods of increasing and decreasing arousal. Each one of us has a window of tolerance or, as it is sometimes called, an *optimal arousal zone*, where we can experience nervous system fluctuations while still having the capacity to regulate ourselves. With a well-regulated nervous system, people only experience extreme highs or lows in their energy and emotions during situations of high stress, danger, or excitement.

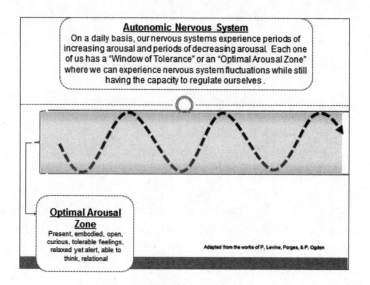

Autonomic Nervous System
On a daily basis, our nervous systems experience periods of increasing arousal and periods of decreasing arousal. Each one of us has a "Window of Tolerance" or an "Optimal Arousal Zone" where we can experience nervous system fluctuations while still having the capacity to regulate ourselves.

Optimal Arousal Zone
Present, embodied, open, curious, tolerable feelings, relaxed yet alert, able to think, relational

Adapted from the works of P. Levine, Porges, & P. Ogden

People with trauma tend to have a poorly regulated nervous system staying in an over- or under-activated state for weeks or months, often getting stuck there. The dysregulation becomes chronic, as they are in a constant state of easily becoming excited, agitated, anxious, tired, or depressed. They are more apt to experience anxiety, panic, difficulty relaxing, restlessness, difficulty sleeping, hostility, chronic low energy, and other such symptoms. They are often in a continuous fluctuation of fight, flight, or freeze responses.

The following visual gives you a portrait of what I think you are experiencing—the emotional roller coaster, the agitation, and the plummet into despair, into the unknown, into the new reality.

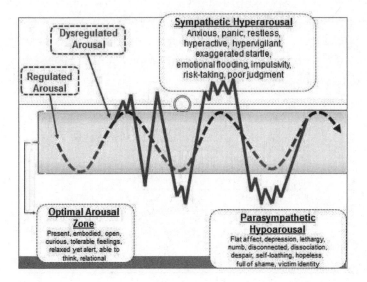

Many of the symptoms that result from chronic gaslighting are the symptoms of post-traumatic stress. Even without gaslighting, the discovery of sexual betrayal can be so traumatic it results in additional symptoms of post-traumatic stress, such as

- Severe anxiety and or panic attacks

- Depression

- Substance abuse

- Inability to focus

- Disturbances in eating and sleeping

- Nightmares

- Intrusive thoughts (flashbacks) or images that are related to information the addict has shared, you witnessed, or inadvertently found

- Preoccupation, rumination

- Hypervigilance

- Lack of sense of safety and security

- Dissociation

- Forms of numbing out, often with alcohol, other drugs, and food

- Severe emotional reactivity

- Self injury

- Suicidal thoughts and or attempts

The depth of trauma does vary for partners. It's influenced by a number of factors.

- Length of time of the deception

- Extent of gaslighting

- Type of acting out (certain sexual acts can be more humiliating and/or shaming)

- Whether or not the sexual behavior is exposed to the public and the ramifications of that

- The degree to which the sexual behavior has impacted finances

- The degree to which the sexual behavior has impacted the children

- If the sexual behavior has had a direct impact on the partners' health

- Previous traumas (If there have been traumas prior to living with sex addiction, and or other acute traumas during this same period of time, the impact has a synergistic effect.)

A factor that can ameliorate the impact of the trauma would be support during the crisis. Unfortunately for most experiencing this crisis, they do so without garnering support of others.

You can heal from this regardless of the depth or breadth of trauma you are experiencing.

Preoccupation and Hypervigilance

Many partners live their lives in response to the addict's behavior. You have this insatiable need to know what your partner is doing, thinking, and feeling so you will know what you are supposed to do, think, or feel. You have suspicions, a sense, a knowing. You wonder; you question. You want to know, but at the same time you don't want to know. You want validation, or you want invalidation. Preoccupation is both a traumatic response and a codependent attribute.

[THERESE]

I don't know how I raised my kids. I was forever distracted. I was always wondering what he was doing, what I could do to be more attractive to him. What was I doing wrong, or what else would he find wrong with me?

[JACQUE]

I would be nice to him when he would come home late, when he would smell of another woman, and when he would blatantly lie to me and I knew it. And then I would go to bed and think of everything I wanted to say to him. I wondered what these other women looked like, what they did together, and what they said to each other. I cannot tell you how many sleepless nights I had.

[MAITE]

I was like a detective checking his calendar, his cell phone account, and his trip schedules for work. I asked pointed questions of his coworkers.

I would set traps for him, not trusting him to act responsibly. And all of the time I certainly felt I had this right.

[PARTNER]

I would drive by where I had heard they met, or drive by her house and look at her to figure out what it was that was so special about her. Even when I had kids, I would load them in the car and go on my searches. I did this with more than one woman and in more than one town as we made several moves across the country.

I snooped in his briefcase, his desk, and his wallet. It was my whole life. And yet I never confronted him.

Hypervigilance becomes a way of life. You vigilantly watch his behavior and try to attach meaning to it. "He came home early, that means . . ." "He's acting all loving, and that means . . ." "He is being nice to the kids, that means . . ." "He's angry, that means . . ." "He's quiet, that means . . ." You may be consumed with what you think he is feeling and thinking. You pride yourself in being able to read his innermost thoughts and feelings. No wonder you are tired, have no time left for yourself, and are losing yourself in the process. You are trying to live inside his body, mind, and heart.

Control

Preoccupation with the addict's problems frequently leads to controlling behavior on your part. Controlling behavior is the manipulation of people, places, and things. It is an attempt to bring stability to chaos and to bring safety to that which is dangerous. Controlling behavior is also a defense against shame. When you are controlling, you don't feel a sense of inadequacy. Instead you feel empowered. At times it's simply an expression of anger. Controlling behavior imparts a sense of power at a time in your life when you are overwhelmed with fear and helplessness. It is a false, hollow power that, at a time of desperation, seems like a quick fix. If you grew up in a physically or emotionally unsafe environment you may also have an already learned response at times of vulnerability. When threatened, you develop survival mechanisms, that is, ways of responding that make it possible to navigate through the pain, the chaos, and the trauma of the moment. At later times in life, you then quickly reengage in that behavior whenever you and the things important to you, such as your relationship, are threatened.

Examples of controlling behavior are:

- Throwing out the stash

  I would find his porn and throw it away. Obviously he knew, but we never talked about it. Maybe that was my way of telling him I knew and therefore believed he would stop.

- Canceling plans

  There were times I'd cancel plans and I would stay home thinking that would make it harder for him to make excuses to go out. Or I thought if I was home he wouldn't get on the internet.

- The silent treatment

  That was my favorite way of punishing him. "I'll show you; I'll just ignore you." He probably liked it, for all I know.

- Relocating

  We moved from one city after another, telling our family it was always for my job or his, as if it were a promotion for us. I was always capitulating to his promises that he would never do it again. We would start over, but nothing ever changed.

- Lying

  I'd lie to him by telling him no one called when I knew that his girlfriend had. I would also lie to him and tell him he had to stay home to be with the kids, and then I would stay at work late on the nights when I was pretty sure they had plans to meet.

- Making threats
  I threatened to tell the kids, tell his parents, tell his boss; to divorce him; to go to her house; and to have my own affairs. My threats were endless.

- Sexual manipulations, such as flirting with others or threatening to be sexual with others to create jealousy in the addict; acting or dressing sexy to gain or maintain his attention; or being sexual with the addict to prevent the addict from being sexual with others
  I pretended I was into certain types of sexual acts that I hated just to try to keep him at home. There were many times I would respond to his sexual advances when I didn't want to or would even initiate sex when I didn't feel sexual, because I thought that if I was sexual enough with him he wouldn't find this need to stray. And looking back, we had a lot of sex, but he had as much if not more with other women. So the truth is he had two stashes: me and the other women.

Controlling behavior is often about what you learned you needed to do to emotionally or even physically survive a threatening situation. While it is ultimately ineffective and self-defeating, don't be judgmental about yourself. Be empathetic to how you got here—from fear, desperation, and shame. Your actions are understandable and natural.

Controlling behaviors rest on the assumption that you have power over the addict. In his book *Contrary to Love: Helping the Sexual Addict*, Patrick Carnes offers an apt analogy: in a traditional African method for trapping monkeys, fruit is placed in small wooden boxes with narrow slats on the sides. The monkeys are able to reach in and grab the fruit but they are unable to pull the fruit out through the slats. Because the monkeys refuse to let go of the fruit, the tribesman can easily capture the monkeys. The monkeys have, in essence, trapped themselves by holding on too tight.[1] This is a metaphor for your plight. You won't let go of control, and so you become imprisoned mistaking control for security.

Image Management

Projecting to the world that you and your family are well and happy reinforces your delusion that everything must be okay. Partners frequently learn to live in fantasy, inventing a false reality that is less painful than the truth. You become adept at living with a high tolerance for inappropriate behavior to the extent that you no longer recognize the inappropriateness. You chronically give the addict the benefit of the doubt; you give away your own reality. You lose yourself in this process, living a life of internal chaos, emotional isolation, and pain marked by control and numbness.

[PARTNER]

I was busy with the kids and my part-time work. We had all of the family toys: a nice home, a nice neighborhood, and vacations once or twice a year. I always had a smile on for the world and even when I was alone I stayed preoccupied with any and everything, truly ignoring the subtle signs. By the time my perfect life was shattered, there had been multiple women, a child he was financially supporting, and job changes that all occurred as a result of his behavior. I just wanted my perfect life where I don't think, don't talk, don't hear, and don't see.

Perfectionism becomes a part of many women's image management. It often stems from internalized shame, operating from the belief that a woman has to be the best to get her partner's or society's approval—or even simply to not be rejected. The belief is this: "If I do more, if I am all things right, everything will be okay."

At some point you learned to push yourself to excel, to be the best. But that means that there is no room for mistakes or vulnerability. Anything less than 150 percent becomes unacceptable. It would mean failure, and there is too much at stake to risk failure. In your mind, not only is your relationship at stake, but also the possible impact on your children, your livelihood, and ultimately your esteem.

[PARTNER]

How could I not act like everything is okay? How could I say to people that my life and my marriage were a farce, a lie? They probably knew, but what did that say about me? I'm a fool? To allow myself to realize I was no different than his previous two wives when I had been so smitten. I was sure he would be different with me. I liked our lifestyle, our friends. I loved him and believed he loved me. So I just kept up the pretense, the image, because to do anything differently would make me question what this meant about me.

Controlling people, places, and things is a part of image management. This external type of control, coupled with a form of internal control where you don't show your feelings or own your needs, is also a part of image management and perfectionism—a cocktail of both trauma response and codependent traits.

For some women, image management is about having a perfectly sculpted body. Many submit to liposuction, cosmetic surgery, and breast augmentation in an attempt to contain the addict's behavior.

[PARTNER]

When I found out about his first affair, I deliberately dieted and decided to have my breasts enlarged. I thought it would please him, but it didn't stop his acting out. I ended up feeling like my body parts were just another part of his addiction.

[PARTNER]

For years he acted out, then one day he left me for good. I was devastated. I went out and had liposuction, Botox, and my breasts lifted. It was as if I wanted to be one of the women he was choosing, yet in reality they didn't look a whole lot different than me. Now I was simply left with a false me.

Having cosmetic surgery is a personal choice, but it is a decision that best comes from a strong sense of self and not from trying to control, sustain, or contain a relationship.

Many women become compulsive about being attractive to their partner. After years and years of being in competition with other women (even if only in fantasy via pornography) and believing you are in constant comparison to other women, the sense of attack on your desirability as a sexual partner wounds your spirit. Adding to this, addicts often lose interest in their partners sexually, as their sexual behavior is not about intimacy. Some women finally give up and become the exact opposite of the firm, gorgeous, made-up woman they were trying to be for their partner. It is not that uncommon for partners to give up on how they look and feel sexually after striving for perfection.

[PARTNER]

In time, I looked the way his rejection made me feel, totally unlovely. It is ironic that pornography and cybersex created the exact opposite in real life of what they must have promised him in his fantasy life.

Distorted Anger

You have the right to be angry; you have reasons to be angry. Anger exists along a continuum, from avoidance to feeling frustrated to blatant rage. Because you are reading this book, you are most likely at one of the ends of the continuum: you are either steely in your outrage with ironclad control or you are fully out of control or perhaps you are completely anger avoidant. You may have moved all over the continuum multiple times. Unfortunately, by now that anger is often both distorted and fueled by myriad other feelings and negative thoughts.

RAGE

"Hell hath no fury like a woman scorned."[2] In the movie *Something to Talk About*, Julia Roberts plays a character who shows up at the local PTA meeting, stands up, and shouts, "Is there anyone here who hasn't slept with my husband?" In the fury of rage you may do things that you never would have imagined yourself doing.

[SARA]

I was hell on wheels and Mt. Vesuvius at the same time. Not a pretty picture. I was ready to string the other women up high. I was most angry when I knew the women, from work or our neighborhood. My husband saw a lot of prostitutes, but I wasn't so angry with them, just him. I guess I thought that is what prostitutes are supposed to do. It is not what a coworker or your neighbor is supposed to do. I would rant and rave at my husband, and he would just stand there most of the time. I think maybe he felt he deserved it. But all it did was offer me a very brief respite and no answers because I had no path, no direction to heal. And my ranting certainly didn't change his behavior.

I would also tell people how awful he was. I once made him bring a coworker to our house so I could yell and rant and rave at her. Another time I went to a motel just to catch him in the act. I was screaming. Oh, I had the anger part down. I was like a spewing volcano, and looking back now I was screaming three generations of women's voices and three generations of anger for betrayal and abandonment—betrayal as the result of substance abuse, sex addiction, suicide, and being untrustworthy.

For some partners, rage is homicidal. Stories of murders and threats are common news. Many years ago Lisa Nowak, an astronaut, drove nine hundred miles with a diaper on so she didn't have to stop en route, totally focused on intending to confront, kidnap, and possibly kill the lover of her lover. Many women do not make the headlines, but their rage is just as destructive. Women have killed or attempted to kill their partners, attempted to throw their partner out of a moving car on the freeway, poisoned their partner's drink or food, sabotaged a partner's parachute, and hired others to commit murder. Sometimes women have burned down their house or removed their partner's belongings and set them on fire. Many betrayed women are empathetic to Lorena Bobbitt's behavior and certainly at least have fantasies of cutting off their partner's penis.

Only a small percentage of betrayed women actually act out their fury violently. More prevalent are homicidal thoughts and moments of fantasy that plot revenge. When you are in a rage, there is a temporary suspension of believing your behavior is wrong. This gives you the perception that what you are doing is defending yourself.

While some people see rage as the behavior of acting out intense and deep anger, I perceive rage as a holding tank, not just for anger, but also for the embarrassment, the humiliations, the fears, and the sadness. Of course you are feeling all of those feelings. There is no doubt you have many reasons to be angry at him: his betrayal of your trust, his disregard for your relationship, the impact of his behaviors on the family and on your health, and the ineffectiveness of loyalty you have shown him in the face of the betrayals. You may be thinking you have wasted a lot of years of your life with him. Or perhaps you are feeling doubly betrayed because of all the years you knew about his behaviors but stayed with him, only to have him walk out once the kids were raised or after you put him through school or after you took care of his sick parents. Maybe your rage comes from feeling trapped, perhaps because you're financially dependent on him or maybe he's your ticket to a green card that allows you to stay in the country or you don't know how you'll raise your kids by yourself. The intensity of your feelings is understandable. The key to greater health is finding the settings in which to express them.

Betrayal hurts. It hurts more deeply than anything you have ever known. But the act of rage will only hurt you in the long run. It's healthier to find something constructive to do with that rage: pound pillows or rip newspapers, scream from the top of a mountain, or write a venomous letter you don't mail. But don't act out your rage toward anyone, including yourself. You deserve better than to act on it and then endure the consequences.

SIDEWAYS ANGER

Often anger becomes sideways or passive-aggressive. Sideways anger occurs when you act it out and then deny it, or you act out in revenge and end up hurting yourself more than him. Your expressions of anger toward the addict can range from threats, screaming, and blaming to giving him the cold shoulder. You may deflect it toward others, often the innocent. In the long run it doesn't make the difference you are hoping for and only creates further chaos.

Here is how the following partners describe their experiences with sideways anger:

- "When I thought he was with a woman, I would get her phone number and call her number incessantly and then hang up."

- "I had an affair to show him."

- "I verbally raged at my kids for things that had nothing to do with them."

- "I spent thousands of dollars shopping when I believed he was lying to me."

- "I keyed his car." (damaging property)

- "I binged on food."

- "I emailed everyone we knew after I discovered emails that told me he was sleeping with a friend. I wanted revenge. I wanted him to be shamed and humiliated. I wanted people to be angry with him and see him as a bad person. In the moment I felt glorious and empowered. But it made no difference other than to scare people away from me in my anger."

- "I would set traps for him in various chat rooms. Sometimes I would surprise him in some humiliating form, but other times I just kept quiet and stored the information to use it as ammunition down the road."

It's so easy to direct blatant or sideways anger toward a third party. You'd rather not hold your partner accountable. It is almost as if the addict is the victim of the situation, victimized by the very person he acts out with. Getting angry with the addict can be threatening to you as you may fear it will push him away when that is not what you want, you really just want him to stop.

[PARTNER]

I spent years being angry with the other women. My husband was a doctor, and in my mind the nurses were always throwing themselves at him. It seemed that every time I became aware of another woman—and they have been in our lives all of our forty years together—I was into another pregnancy or had my own health problem. The timing was such that I thought I needed him, and that meant being angry with someone other than him. Besides, if I got angry with him, maybe that would push him more toward them.

[SARA]

Most of the time my anger was with my husband unless I knew the other woman. Then it was as if I thought she had assaulted him and he had no part in it. I would switch my emotional alliances back and forth between my husband and the woman, seeing one as the victim of the other.

ANGER AVOIDANCE
Reactivity on the part of partners can be identified as a fight or flight response. When it comes to anger, blatant rage is clearly the fight, and sideways anger a more subtle form of fight. A flight response is often demonstrated when searching for a way to medicate your pain, often through food, alcohol or other drugs, or some form of behavior that allows you disconnection. If you find yourself incapable of feeling angry, feeling more a sense of defeat or numbness, you are in a freeze reaction.

Some partners say they just don't feel angry; instead they feel defeated or numb. They may acknowledge that they *should* feel angry but aren't. For many women, avoidance is a learned response to stress over time; a response that is often acquired in childhood and/or as the consequence of long-term hurtful adult relationships. It is often a part of low-grade chronic depression (dysthymia) or major depression. You may have learned that by responding to a bad situation with judicious anger you didn't change the predicament; you only felt helpless. When anger doesn't restore your sense of control over the environment you eventually begin to feel apathetic; you come to believe that nothing good will ever come of it, so why expend the energy to just feel more battered?

You may be using the distraction of busyness to help stuff your anger. Busyness is often demonstrated through housework, shuffling kids to activities and appointments, shopping, or work. Some women act out their busyness by getting overly involved in the community. It could mean that you spend hours at the health club or on the computer. By themselves none of these behaviors are bad, and in fact they are often esteemed. But for the partner, involvement that is excessive, that is done in a way to avoid the issues in your relationship and family, merely serves as an unhealthy diversion.

[PARTNER]

I became like a spinning top. I had myself so busy with kids, work, parents—anything to avoid the reality. I didn't know what to do. I didn't want to lose him. So I just kept my mouth shut and dug my head into my work, my career.

Rage and sideways anger can provide fleeting moments of revenge or personal satisfaction. However, in the end they, or the acts of anger avoidance, only lessen your self-respect, dignity, and self-esteem. The potential fallout and consequences can be devastating.

Chronic Grief and Loss

Loss of what you have hoped and worked for in intimacy, loss of the way you know yourself and your partner, loss regarding the way you think about people and the world you live in, and/or loss of a relationship—whatever it is that is gone or has now changed in your life will generate all of the basic stages in the grief process.[3] Initial shock, disbelief, denial, anger, guilt and bargaining, despair, loneliness, and acceptance are natural responses to any loss. Losing a loved one to addiction has the potential of keeping you stuck in the process of grief because the addict has not died; he is still present and his acting out continues. Living with addiction and reacting to addiction causes you to live in a chronic state of loss. You feel the loss, go in and out of denial, experience anger and guilt, attempt to bargain, feel despair, and at times are lifted by hope. Partners may live for years caught up in the cycle of chronic grief and all of its many feelings. Your losses are ongoing and repetitive with denial entering and leaving the picture. Not having the truth validated, discounting your own perceptions or having them dismissed by others, and minimizing feelings all lead to a distorted and unmanageable internal life.[3]

In the throes of living with addiction, you may spend more time processing one aspect of grief than another. It's only natural that you stay in the stage that is familiar or safe. If anger is a haven because you feel empowered by it, you might go there and get stuck. If you are anger avoidant and you have taken on a lot of guilt in your life, you may readily go there. Guilt and bargaining frequently work together, causing you to make statements like "If I_____, he will_____." "If I pay more sexual attention to him, he will not stray. If I am the perfect wife, he will never leave me." You may refuse to accept reality, become angry and blaming, and keep trying to bargain with the addict. "I'll move anywhere you want.

We can change churches. I will change my job. I will do whatever will make you happier so you will stop this behavior." You may get stuck in sorrow, feeling the pain, hurt, and sadness, but you don't find a way out of it. In defeat, you succumb to depression. To compound the tragedy, you may engage in actions that are self-degrading, self-destructive, or that profoundly violate your own values.

While you are stuck in your grief, you go through a wide range of feelings about the addict as you increasingly suspect or become aware of the behavior. Feelings fluctuate wildly, from intense rage to profound sadness, fear, embarrassment, shame, and guilt. You may keep these feelings tightly controlled and to yourself or they may leak everywhere. You may be out grocery shopping and when someone bumps into your cart you react as if the person has just stolen your child. A casual conversation with an acquaintance who simply asks you how you are, not knowing what is happening in your life, sends you into inconsolable grief and you end up spilling your guts.

So what do you do to cope with your grief? Your responses probably run the gamut.

At times of great fear, angst, and shame, women employ a variety of disconnection strategies: they move toward, move against, or move away.

- In moving *toward* you seek to appease and please, you become Ms. Perfect, Ms. Accommodator.

- In moving *against* you act aggressively to garner power. You can do this with rageful or spiteful behavior. You may engage in your own acting out via self-destructive behaviors, such as using drugs, having affairs, or spending money.

- In moving away you withdraw, hide, silence yourself, and keep secrets. You numb out or slip into depression and anxiety. Overeating, anorexic behavior, and the use of alcohol or other drugs (particularly sedatives or depressants) also aid in withdrawing and hiding.

Most people relate to using all three or a combination of strategies. None of these movements help; they keep you stuck. They are all self- defeating.

Which of the above do you engage in?

[PARTNER]

In the early years of my marriage I bent over backward to be the accommodating wife. I suspected he was with other women, yet I felt trapped financially. I was scared to leave, scared to be on my own. I was scared the kids would blame me because they wouldn't understand why I wanted to leave. In time I started to secretly drink and then use pills. I felt so defeated. I just wanted to disappear but couldn't. I got so preoccupied with my suspicions, and yet felt so defeated, so I sent threatening letters to the women I suspected he was with and damaged the possessions he seemed so fond of, such as his musical instruments and his car.

The Body Knows

One of the consequences of not acknowledging your feelings is the real possibility of health problems. Your autoimmune system can become severely compromised when you are undergoing emotional stress.

[PARTNERS]

After a few months in recovery, I was able to see how much I rationalized my feelings away and rationalized my trust in my husband. But by this time I was in a chronic state of physical pain. I had been going to doctors for the past couple of years and had a host of different tests. I was just given many different diagnoses and medical suggestions. Then I got into recovery and realized I hadn't seen a doctor in over two months, then three months, and then four months. Today I don't run from conflict. Today I know when I am angry. Today I don't keep that stupid smile on my face like all is fine with the world when I really feel as if my world is crumbling.

Today I have no mysterious physical pains.

Whether you know for sure that your partner is acting out sexually or not, you are living with stress. You are dealing with both acute stress and a more subtle chronic state of stress. Living with the fears of what it may mean to your marriage and your family if you acknowledge the sex addiction, and living with the suspicion that something is off in your marriage but not knowing exactly what, are both anxiety provoking. This stress is traumatic to your body. While you may normalize, minimize, and rationalize something in your mind, the physical body knows something is wrong. When it's in jeopardy, be it physical or psychological jeopardy, the body mobilizes its defenses. Stress can trigger the body's response to perceived threat or danger, called the *fight or flight response*, which generates the release of certain hormones such as adrenaline and cortisol that speed the heart rate, slow digestion, shunt blood flow to major muscle groups, and change various other autonomic nervous functions, giving the body a burst of energy and strength. Originally named for its ability to enable us to physically fight or run away when faced with danger, this response is now activated in situations where neither response is appropriate, like during a stressful day at work or at home. When the perceived threat is gone, our bodily systems and chemistry are designed to return to normal function via the relaxation response, but in a state of chronic stress, this adjustment often doesn't happen enough, causing damage to the body. When a machine is operated at maximum speed, the sustained high speed pushes the mechanisms past their limits or begins to burn out the elements. Our bodies and minds will react the same way. When pushed past their limits, they begin to break down. Pretty soon things start to fall apart. In this process, as a consequence of our stress, the autoimmune capacity is lower, rendering us more vulnerable to illness.

THE IMPACT OF STRESS

Critical factors that affect the impact of stress are twofold: how far your system is taxed and for how long. Some stressors may occur only once or a few times but their impact is so great that trauma takes hold. Rape, an accident, or an assault may fit this form of trauma. Other trauma experiences may be less acute, but they happen every day and the hurt accumulates. In a coupleship, little acts of degradation, manipulation, secrecy, and shame on a daily basis take their toll. The body knows.

Many cognitive conditions are caused or exacerbated by stress. They include:

- poor memory
- seeing only the negative
- indecisiveness
- anxious or racing thoughts
- inability to concentrate
- constant worrying
- trouble thinking clearly
- loss of objectivity
- poor judgment
- dread

Common illnesses and physical symptoms associated with stress are:

- headaches or backaches
- diarrhea or constipation
- nausea
- dizziness, fatigue

- insomnia
- frequent colds or flu
- grinding teeth

- chest pain
- rapid heart rate
- ulcers
- hair loss
- depression
- diabetes
- hyperthyroidism
- rheumatoid arthritis

- weight gain or loss
- shortness of breath
- skin breakouts (hives, eczema)
- high blood pressure
- chronic back pain
- sleep disturbance
- sweats
- anxiety disorder
- heart disease
- tooth and gum disease
- asthma

[MAITE]

Today when I have sleep problems or when a headache begins or when my back begins to hurt, I know it can be something organic, but knowing what I know about me, I use it as a warning that I may be in over my head with stress. Usually these things happen when I am neglecting myself, not taking time for myself, eating poorly, or have not done any exercise in months. Clearly I am ignoring my feelings. I see it as a symptom that I am not doing what I need to do.

[PARTNER]

At the height of the insanity I'd experience as many as seven facial tics in rapid succession. They began as small twitches near my eyes; then they expanded to include more twitches in my cheeks and around my mouth. This phenomenon continued for years, abating and increasing with tension and stress. I felt I must look like a contortionist. After I separated from my husband and began living alone, all such symptoms disappeared. In the past years, when under stress, I have been aware of some less intense twitching. When I became quite stressed while witnessing my daughter during her divorce proceedings, ending a very abusive marriage to an alcoholic, I noticed my face twitching again. I think I was thrown into a memory pool and began swimming in my own situation again. For now, I am tic free and hope to keep stress at a manageable level.

[PARTNER]

I don't know what caused my fibromyalgia, but now that I'm in recovery I no longer experience the physical pain or incredible fatigue that I once did. I can now do all kinds of things that I wasn't able to do previously. I can get up, get dressed, and go out; I can drive again, and I'm not depressed. Is my being in recovery helping to diminish the pain of my fibromyalgia? Is one connected to the other? I don't know, but I'm not going to give up my recovery to find out. I believe I am in remission because I now have a voice and no longer accept being bullied, and I no longer doubt myself. It's like my body was forsaken by my heart and soul and once I began to honor me, my body began coming back to health.

When faced with chronic stress and an overactivated autonomic nervous system, people begin to experience physical symptoms.

The first symptoms are relatively mild, like chronic headaches and increased susceptibility to colds. With more exposure to chronic stress, however, more serious health problems may develop. Stress has the ability to worsen many diseases that may be caused by other factors.

STRESS AND SERIOUS ILLNESS

Today medical researchers certainly recognize the role stress plays as a contributor to cancers. It's believed by many medical professionals that stress weakens the immune system, significantly reducing the body's number of T cells, which are responsible for defending against malignant cancer cells. The T cells in the immune system are the body's only real means of defending itself against cancer cells, and they can only be created during the body's relaxation cycle.

Two Women of the Lodge have been challenged by cancer. They both believe their recovery from their trauma decreased their stress and heightened their physical well-being.

[VANESSA]

As my husband and I began recovery, I was diagnosed with aggressive ovarian cancer. When presented with a scenario like this, the medical community is anxious to label it as genetic. I'm sure genes do play a role in it, but I also strongly believe that my family's inheritance of cancer has been related to the fact that we all operated from the ingrained belief that emotional suppression equaled survival. We bottled and stuffed anything that wasn't happy. You can't keep pushing every negative feeling and event into dark places in your soul and not expect them to have an impact. I never learned to deal with painful situations in a healthy way, so I believe my body was storing those memories at a cellular level, which would later manifest as cancer.

There is no question in my mind that much more than genes contributed to my cancer. I had suffered severe emotional abuse from a very young age. Keeping secrets set the framework for emotional suppression and abuse to become the foundation of my psyche. I held myself and those around me to perfectionist, unrealistic standards. I led an incredibly stressful lifestyle. I was a work addict and had very intense, high-pressure jobs and always pushed myself to higher levels of achievement. I was dealing with the ongoing and progressive infidelity of my husband, and my own raging codependent behaviors, and I was doing so much for others that I was putting basic self-care at the bottom of the list.

I also believe that much more than chemotherapy contributed to healing from my cancer. When I was diagnosed, the cancer had already moved into my liver. The prognosis was grim. I defied the odds and am now deemed a medical anomaly—or miracle, depending on the circle. I believe this was achieved through approaching my healing on many levels. I worked with every medical modality—traditional oncology, Ayurvedic, Chinese, alternative, holistic, and naturopathic—and I changed my diet and fitness.

I engaged in the deepest therapy available to address the many suppressed areas of my life. I had strong mentorship and support groups. An amazing network of people rallied around me and gave me the strength to do all this incredibly hard work while fighting for my life. Rigorous purging of the old traumas, rethinking accountability, and owning my own issues and negative messages were key elements. This multi-layered work continues to occur, though less intensively, on an ongoing basis. I believe all of it was integral to my healing and ultimately focused me on authenticity and self-love.

The combination of all these things saved my life and gave me the strength to make healthier choices. My perspective on most everything has changed, and now I try to live from a place of making the most of every day.

[SARA]

I know that my concern, anger, stress, and living with addictive behaviors were the enemies of my immune system. My survival instincts were strong, too. I asked for an MRI for some reason, and it found the cancer cells years before they would have been discovered by mammography or other standard diagnostic tests. This instinctive stand for my own life and health was a true paradigm shift for me. I turned forward and began the process of setting boundaries around the respect I had for my life and my value. It works both ways. While I believe my lifestyle compromised my immune system, my willingness to hear my inner voice and trust myself got me to a diagnosis and treatment at an early stage. Then embracing life and health drove my desire for recovery—to live life in truth—my truth with integrity. It's been ten years now, and I've never been healthier in mind, body, and spirit.

Clearly chronic stress has a strong impact on the immune system, particularly one that is already compromised. Learning how to take care of yourself in recovery will help you to relieve stress.

Behavioral Health Issues

ADDICTION: SUBSTANCE AND PROCESS

It is not uncommon that as a response to stress and as a means to manage intolerable feelings, a betrayed partner finds herself engaging in and depending upon addictive behaviors. It may be a substance addiction found in the use of alcohol or other drugs. Often it is a process or behavioral addiction. Food is a particularly strong anesthetizer for women. Anorexia and bulimia with themes of control and image management are pervasive and common. Frequently, partners identify with compulsive spending or shopping. Some partners find solace in gambling or online gaming. It is also possible that any sexual acting out on your part may be addictive. You may find yourself relying more and more on the use of these manifestations to help you cope with the stress of the betrayal. Complicating the situation, many partners will come to identify with relationship and love addiction, often within the coupleship making it difficult to engage in recovery practice due to unhealthy bonding to the person acting out.

Today we know that as far as the brain is concerned a reward is a reward, regardless of whether it comes from a substance, behavior, or experience. Love and relationship addicted patterns may occur, and these are shaped by an underlying belief that your worth and value are measured through your relationship with a partner regardless of how he or she treats you.

We live in a quick fix, feel good culture that reinforces seeking outside answers to inside problems. While it may be your partner's behavior that led you to read this book, this is also the time for your own self-exploration.

The behaviors may have preceded the sexual addiction in your coupleship or they may be an adaptive response to this crisis. It's important to recognize being addicted is not a statement about your worth or value, nor does it reflect a lack of strength or willpower. It does not in any capacity lessen the impact that your partner's sexual betrayal has on you and your relationship.

SAFE

A simple way to think about whether or not something is a problem for you is using the acronym of SAFE:

- **S** stands for secretive. Is the behavior, the substance, the frequency, or the amount in which you engage something others are not aware of? Is it something you do not want to discuss openly? You may think it is not a secret, but in fact, if you find you're not being open about the degree to which you spend time engaging in or are preoccupied with it, then it is secretive.

- **A** stands for abusive. Is the behavior or substances hurtful or harmful to yourself or another at this stage? Is it hurting your relationship with someone else even if he or she is unaware? Is it harming you in some way, keeping you away from other priorities? Is it harmful to your self-esteem? Your finances? Your health?

- **F** stands for feelings. Does this process or behavior separate or remove you from your feelings? Does it medicate your feelings? Or is it the only time in which you experience feelings?

- **E** stands for emptiness. After you have engaged in this process or behavior for some time, does it now leave you with a sense of emptiness? Do you find yourself reengaging more quickly than you have in the past—leading to another **E,** which is escalation.

If you identify with any of the four letters I encourage you to share what is happening for you with a trusted person, but if you identify with all four letters associated with SAFE, I strongly encourage you to see a professional.

MOOD AND ANXIETY DISORDERS

Both depression and various forms of anxiety are common for partners. While people who struggle with these issues often have a biological predisposition, repeated psychological injury and chronic stress is a major contributor to both. The accumulation of loss that occurs when you are in a relationship with an addict also fuels a level of grief where depression becomes a consequence to unattended sorrow. And certainly living in a constant state of biological alert and hypo-arousal will create anxiety. Both depression and anxiety are most often trauma responses. Upon a thorough assessment by a healthcare professional, it may be helpful to include medication as another tool to help you in your recovery process. Do be aware that the use of any mood-altering substance may aggravate and mask symptoms of anxiety or depressive disorders.

* * *

In a healing journey you will learn how to stand tall in the face of truth. Standing tall means finding the voice to speak your truth, knowing and honoring your needs and feelings, and having boundaries that offer both containment and protection. This takes work on your part, but as you are reading this book, it is possible, particularly with the support of other women who have made this journey before you. You lose sight of your true self when you act out in emotional pain. The good news is that there is a path out of the pain; you can live your life differently.

Reflective Thoughts and Questions

- Give three examples of your denial process.

- Name three rationalizations and minimizations you most identify with.

- Can you identify with having been gaslighted and the consequences of it?

- Can you see your emotional dysregulation as portrayed in the visuals presented?

- To what degree do you struggle with Post-Traumatic Stress?

- Have you been preoccupied by the addict's behavior?

- In what ways have you attempted to control the addict's behavior?

- Has maintaining an image been important to you? If so, describe how you've been presenting yourself and what it's been covering up.

- Would you describe yourself as perfectionistic? If so, describe your perfectionistic thoughts and behaviors, and then identify what you think fuels this behavior.

- Describe your anger. Have you felt or acted out in fury or rage? Is your anger a sideways anger? How have you expressed it?

- Where do you see yourself in the grief process?

- In what ways has your body been speaking to you?

- Are you aware of any behaviors that could be an addiction for you? Identify and explain your thoughts and concerns. Are you willing to seek help to assess this?

- If you are struggling with depression and anxiety would it be helpful to have your anxiety and depression assessed for possible medication intervention?

- What was important for you to learn in this chapter?

CHAPTER TWO NOTES

1   Patrick Carnes, *Contrary to Love: Helping the Sexual Addict* (Center City, MN: Hazelden, 1994).

2   Adaptation of the closing line of Act III of *The Mourning Bride* by William Congreve, first produced in 1697: "Heav'n has no rage, like love to hatred turn'd. Nor Hell a fury, like a woman scorn'd."

3   Elisabeth Kübler-Ross, *On Death and Dying* (New York: Simon & Schuster, 1997).

CHAPTER THREE

His Behavior Is Not About You

Why is he doing this?

Why won't he just stop?

First and foremost, you need to know that his behavior is not about you. As hurtful as his behavior is, he isn't doing this deliberately to hurt you or to punish you. Regardless of what he may say, he is not doing this because of anything you have done or not done, the way you look or don't look. It is not willfulness on his part. He has reached a stage where he cannot stop acting out sexually without help.

However you describe what it is you are living with, it is very important to see the addictive aspect of your partner's behavior. I know some readers have already had negative reactions to identifying the betrayal in their coupleship as sex addiction. Having been shaped by social, cultural, and religious beliefs the meaning we attach to sex and sexuality varies from individual to individual.

Family values and behaviors may have the greatest impact. The same is true of the word addiction, and its myriad implications and judgments. As a result, it is not uncommon for some people to find the words "sex addiction" offensive or frightening. Perhaps you also think that by viewing or naming it as addiction, it lets your partner off the hook for his behavior. Absolutely not, the addict is responsible for his recovery and that includes accountability.

Historically, the term addiction was first identified as the out-of-control use of alcohol and other drugs. Today, we recognize that many behaviors—gambling, eating, internet, shopping, and/or engaging in sex—can spin out of control and become addictive.

Just as alcoholism has existed over the centuries, using sex in a compulsive, addictive manner has also been occurring for many generations. The Italian-born libertine Giacomo Casanova was such a famous womanizer that, a full two centuries after his death, his name remains synonymous with the art of seduction. Benjamin Franklin is believed to have abandoned his devoted wife, Deborah, and became a lecher in London and France. In his book *The Autobiography of Benjamin Franklin*, Mr. Franklin confessed that as a young man, his "hard-to-govern'd passion of youth" led him into intrigues with women.[1] It is said he went to women hungrily, secretly, and briefly. Wilt Chamberlain, famous professional basketball player, devoted an entire chapter of his autobiography to his sexual exploits. He said that if he had to count his sexual encounters, he would be closing in on 20,000 women. "Yes, that's correct, twenty thousand different ladies," he wrote. "At my age, that equals out to having sex with 1.2 women a day, every day since I was fifteen years old."[2] Historically, this kind of behavior by men has been normalized by our society and in many cultures continues to be accepted. As a consequence of the #MeToo movement, sexual assaults, harassment, and sexual exploits and secrets of men not only are not being tolerated, they are much more apt to be exposed and reported.

Whether or not your partner's behavior is ultimately diagnosed as addictive, you and he both deserve the opportunity to seek professional help. You can still find a path for yourself as you understand your own role in this partnership and a path out of your angst and despair.

The Addiction

Sexually addictive behavior is an equal opportunity addiction that spans all boundaries: economic, political, gender, sexual orientation, intellectual, religious, racial, and ethnic. Sex addicts come from all walks of life: they are factory workers, salespeople, truck drivers, janitors, policemen, accountants, physicians, politicians, executives, and clergy members. Most people who act out sexually during their adult years were abused sexually, physically, or emotionally during their childhood. The majority grew up in families where addiction already flourished. Many grapple with other forms of addiction in addition to their sexual compulsivity.

Addiction is not about a particular behavior but its overall context. Just as there is a distinction between the social drinker and the alcoholic, there is a distinction between the person who has one affair and the person who repeatedly has affairs even when a job or marriage may be in jeopardy. Not everyone who has affairs, participates in unsafe sex, or keeps sexual secrets is a sex addict. Not everyone who views pornography, engages in anonymous sex, visits prostitutes, or performs acts of bondage/dominance or sadomasochism is a sex addict. The type of sexual activity one prefers, the choice of sexual partners, or where one goes to have sex does not determine sex addiction. When a person deviates from the established sexual norms it does not make him a bad person, nor does it mean he is addicted.

The elements that define sexual addiction are the compulsive nature of the experience, the repetition of the behavior despite its negative consequences, the need for more and more to achieve the same effect, and the bad feelings that it engenders. The escalation in the amount of sexual activity or intensity of the experience occurs because the current level no longer provides the fix it once did. An addict has a persistent pursuit of self- destructive or high-risk sexual behavior, wherein cherished aspects of one's life are potentially sacrificed.

[ADDICT]

At times I would tell myself this is it, no more. But that never lasted for long. I would again find myself acting out. I didn't see it as acting out. I was just still doing what I had been doing, be it an affair, pornography, or a massage parlor. I would totally forget that I had a moment of thinking I shouldn't be doing this. The truth is, most of the time I just didn't see it as something I needed to stop. I was so caught up in just me or my next conquest. It was like I felt I was entitled to this life. If I were to think about it, I just totally separated it from my relationship with my wife. Today I know that is hard to grasp, but that is what I was thinking during the behavior. My behavior had nothing to do with my marriage, nothing to do with my wife. It was about me. I would have been doing this no matter who I was married to.

While an accepted definition of addiction is "a pathological relationship with a mood-altering chemical," the American Psychiatric Association (APA) offers a more clinical definition: "Addiction is a complex condition, a brain disease that is manifested by compulsive substance use despite harmful consequence. People with addiction (severe substance use disorder) have an intense focus on using a certain substance(s), such as alcohol or drugs, to the point that it takes over their life." The addict's relationship with the substance of choice becomes more important to him or her than family, friends, health, or work, and it progresses to the point where consumption and/or use are necessary to feel normal.

In order to feel adequate, the addict comes to depend on a change in neurochemistry and the accompanying mood-altering experience; it becomes central to his or her life. The vow to stop the behaviors gets lost against the power of the addiction. All of that is equally true for the sex addict.

THE BEHAVIORS

As a drug addict may use pain medications, heroin, and marijuana, sexually compulsive people often engage in a combination of behaviors. The behaviors can range from pornography, to one-night affairs and long-term relationships. He may engage with prostitutes (escorts), massage parlor workers, or in chat rooms on the internet. Some sex addicts are drawn to voyeurism, exhibitionism, or connecting sexually with someone of the same gender when one is not gay.

People who are acting out sexually find the internet exacerbates their problem. Even if someone has not previously been acting out, internet access to pornography and cybersex often incites escalating and provocative behavior. It also contributes to acting out in real life. Online sexual behavior has been described as the "crack cocaine of sex addiction" because of its accessibility and affordability. Just pushing a button gives a person access to his secret world. He doesn't have to go to outside of the home or office, put himself at physical risk, or cruise the streets. Anytime, day or night, in the comfort of his home or workplace, his fix is available with devastating consequences just as harmful as real-time sex addiction.

Just as the majority of alcoholics are not homeless, most sex addicts do not fit the erroneous stereotype of criminal offenders who satisfy their needs by forcing themselves on helpless victims. This is not to say that there are not victims in sexual addiction. In reality, all addictive sexual behavior is victimizing; the addict and his partner are both hurt in the process. The behaviors of a sex addict are often emotionally hurtful and disrespectful of others, but only a few behaviors are considered crimes and those differ in the degree of personal violence involved. Certainly, child molestation and rape inflicts deep emotional wounds, but many people who commit sex crimes, specifically child molesters and rapists, are not compulsive. They are sociopaths engaged in acts of aggression. Sexually addictive behavior does not necessarily indicate criminal behavior; likewise, committing sexual crimes does not necessarily indicate sex addiction.

Research in the field of addiction supports the belief that different forms of addiction taps into the same brain chemistry.[3] Today we recognize there are three different types of addiction: 1) arousal, 2) satiation, and 3) fantasy. Whatever the substance or behavior, it can manifest in any one of these types.

Arousal-type addictions are also thought of as intensity addictions; the sex addict is hooked on the rush that occurs with risky sexual activities— the combination of fear and danger. The danger can be physical danger or a social danger, such as being caught in the act. Satiation-type addictions are seen in behaviors that medicate personal pain and anxiety. Fantasy-type addictions involve imagined sexual experiences.

Many addicts mix and match their sexually addictive behaviors as well as other addictive disorders. One can move from fantasy and escape to arousal and back to escape. For example, a man who masturbates while fantasizing he is having sex with a woman he sees on the internet. Then at greater risk to himself, he moves on to meeting this woman in person and after having a clandestine meeting of rough sex he returns home to a night of drinking to oblivion.

Addicts live an all-or-nothing kind of life, not knowing how to moderate themselves. They know two ways: full-out high speed or full-on brakes. Intensity addicts who are more apt to engage in high-risk dangerous situations commonly engage in satiation fixes to calm down and soothe their heightened energy, enabling them to be able to resume normal activities.

[ADDICT]

My father raged and was abusive. By age eleven I found what my father had—power in raging. It protected me from my fears, my sense of unworthiness. Then I discovered masturbation and it calmed me. It was a solace.

Rage gave me the high, the power, and masturbation was my anesthetic. They worked in tandem for years.

Because a sex addict is a person who never learned to tolerate his painful feelings, he seeks escape from those feelings. Sexual activity and sexual fantasy alter brain chemistry in the same way by producing profound feelings of pleasure. Sex addicts are altering their brain chemistry, and as a result, their mood, all the time. They use sex as a drug to produce a high. As his disease progresses, the sex addict cares less and less who his sexual partner is. If he can't find a partner, masturbation will give him a quick fix. His chief pursuit is the high.

THE SCIENCE OF ADDICTION

While a nonaddicted individual can quickly see how the addict's behavior causes problems or has the potential to do so, the addicted person continues the behaviors despite the risks. He either doesn't recognize the impact his behavior is having on his committed relationship or he is willing to risk the relationship. He may lose jobs, put himself (as well as his loved ones) at high risk for sexually transmitted diseases, and be willing to risk lawsuits or experience bankruptcy, all while downplaying these possibilities.

[ADDICT]

I think back about my behavior. There was so much deception, lying, working the room. There was no turning it on or off. I really thought it was okay. I was clueless to the damage. I rationalized my first divorce not being about my behavior but that she just wanted different things. Today I am stunned at my own thinking, or lack of thinking, back then.

[ADDICT]

I didn't know how to stop. It sounds so strange, but until I got help I didn't realize that it was truly an addiction for me. I was incapable of stopping on my own. I needed help. Left to my own thinking, I thought I had my life in control. The twisted thinking here is that I thought I had all of my lies covered and that meant all was okay.

The science of addiction indicates that the inability to recognize the impact of behavior on others or the willingness to risk what is significant in one's life appears to be connected to brain chemistry. How many times have you said or wanted to say to your partner, "What are you thinking?" The answer is: he is not thinking.

When people use substances or engage in escape behaviors, the brain releases neurotransmitters, such as adrenaline and dopamine, that trigger the brain's pleasure/reward center; or it may release serotonin, which lessens anxiety and depression. With repetitive engagement, the triggers in the brain's reward center override the cognitive, rational thinking part of the brain. Brain scans show there are reduced levels of activation in the prefrontal cortex, where rational thought should be able to override impulsive behavior. But under the influence, it doesn't. The prefrontal cortex succumbs to the limbic system, the emotional, reactive area of the brain. In essence, addiction is a hijacked brain.

Addiction is not about substances or behaviors, but is about disrupting the processing of pleasure; the balance point is shifted so you keep creating more and more urges, and you keep wanting more and more.

Science also tells us that stress alters the way we think. Parts of the brain that help us problem-solve shut down at times of stress, fueling impulsive behavior. When this behavior becomes excessive, the brain interprets the feelings as positive and cannot recognize the long-term consequences, telling us "this is good; we should do it again."

The good news in looking at the science is to know that the brain has plasticity to it. That means the practices people learn in treatment and in recovery affect brain function in a positive manner. An addict can learn skills to calm the emotionally reactive area of the brain, avoid triggers that activate the emotional area, and enhance the decision-making area where he can rationally think through his decisions, rather than responding impulsively and from such a strong emotional basis.

THE ADDICTIVE CYCLE

Being addicted means that at some point a person loses the ability to choose whether or not he is going to be sexual. He is unable to say no to his impulses and cravings. Be it alcohol, gambling, or sex, the addicted person either doesn't see it or denies the problems that his compulsive activity is continuously producing in his life, maintaining his denial with rationalizations. Sex addicts are preoccupied with and compulsive about their sexuality. They engage in distorted thinking, rationalizing, and defending and justifying their behavior while blaming others for the problems that result. Like those addicted to alcohol and/or other drugs, sex addicts progress through stages in which they retreat further and further from the reality of friends, family, and work, and potentially destroy those important relationships, sabotage careers, and risk significant health issues and violent death.

Sex addicts describe their euphoria with sex similarly to that described by drug addicts with drug use. This may be an effect of endorphins and other endogenous brain chemicals that are excited during sexual behaviors, creating a drug-induced state. The mood-altering experience is not just the sexual act itself; it can be produced by sexual fantasy and rituals as well.

Patrick Carnes, PhD, a pioneer in the sex addiction field, delineated key components of the addictive cycle as it relates to sexual compulsivity.[4] Obsession and preoccupation are the thinking disorder aspects of addiction. People can become obsessive about any activity that generates a positive mood for them, whether it is the self-nurturing feeling of eating, the excitement of gambling, or the arousal of seduction. Addicts find that just thinking about a sexual act leads to a preoccupation that in itself produces pleasurable and exciting sensations, creating a positive mood in order to avoid a negative one. It can be employed at any time of the day in any situation. Often sex addicts seem as though they are not present even when they are physically there. Their mental arousal makes them less and less in tune with the emotional stresses that triggered the fantasy and creates a pressing desire to act out their thoughts. The fantasy, the anticipation, the planning, and the risk-taking are as important as the sexual act itself. For some addicts, the thinking about, planning of, and anticipation of the behavior is the most pleasurable part of their addictive cycle. As the addict moves into fantasy, his neurochemistry begins to unleash the chemicals that an actual sexual encounter would prompt. Spurred to action by sexual fantasies, the addict begins to prepare for sexually acting out.

[ADDICT]

My actual sexual indiscretion was only minutes, but the planning and anticipating took hours.

> I couldn't even remember things about my job or what was happening at home. I was mentally consumed with the fantasy or was covering my bases and finessing my lies.

Engaging in pre-sexual rituals intensifies the powerful emotional and neurochemical high and drives the addictive cycle forward. Rituals are as varied in number and complexity as there are sex addicts. Some rituals may take minutes, others hours. Some sex addicts will travel great distances to obtain pornography and won't act out until they return home. Some will make elaborate travel plans in order to connect with partners from around the country or the world. The ritual might include changing into erotic clothing, listening to specific music, cruising by car in a favorite neighborhood, or going online. For some, the ritual involves the use of alcohol or other drugs. Just like fantasies in the preoccupation stage, rituals produce excitement. Perhaps the excitement comes from anticipating going to a massage parlor that practices techniques the addict hasn't experienced before. Maybe the excitement is produced by the amount of risk involved in a certain activity. Danger and intrigue are exciting to the addict and summon the release of adrenaline, which is in itself is addictive. Through the preoccupation and ritual stages, the addict's brain has literally created a chemical cocktail that is as addictive as any drug. Any addictive behavior can be dangerously pursued and therefore is exciting, giving addicts a rush.

Once addicts have reached their ritual stage, it is almost inevitable that they will go on to the acting-out stage. Moments, hours, or even days into their fantasies and rituals, sex addicts arrive at the full-blown expression of their sexual behavior. Compulsive masturbation with pornography, exhibitionism, voyeurism, hiring of prostitutes, paying for sexual massages, and visiting sex clubs are intensely stimulating.

Once he has acted out, he may or may not look back with regret, fear, or anxiety about what he has been doing sexually or otherwise. He may suffer direct unwanted consequences as a result of his sexual conduct, which makes him feel even worse. Since addicts act out in part to compensate for their limited emotional coping skills, their sexual behavior and its consequences often make them feel worse about themselves over time, which in turn causes an escalation of the frequency and intensity of their behaviors. They lose faith in themselves and turn more frequently to sex to try to feel better. The depression, shame, and anxiety generated by their sexual acting out can bring addicts back to the very need for emotional control that initiated the addiction cycle at the outset. Each addict has his own particular response to his behavior and his unique way of gearing up for the next time. Think of a merry-go-round in motion; it is difficult to get off.

All addiction is characterized as progressive with diminishing returns, meaning there is a need for more of the chemical or more of the compulsive activity to get the same level of satisfaction. Over time, alcoholics require more and more alcohol in order to feel good. Likewise, the sex addict will find himself taking more and greater risks in order to feel the same level of excitement. Early in his addiction, an addict establishes rules that allow him to believe he has control over his behavior. While addiction serves its purpose to anesthetize an inner shame, to offer a false esteem, or even to produce feelings of power or control, the addict is certainly not delusional in his thinking all the time. There are times when he is aware of his dishonesty, ashamed of his lies, and feels guilty for the pain he is causing his partner. It is then that he tells himself he won't do it again or he puts restrictions on himself. He often promises himself he will do things differently next time, and then he feels twice as bad when he cannot keep his promises. As the alcoholic tries to control his behavior by saying to himself he will only drink after a certain hour or only on weekends or only certain liquor, people who are sexually addicted impose their own restrictions (as seen in the examples below) and soon break their own rules:

- "I will only engage with prostitutes when I am on business out of town, never in my own city."

- "I will only have affairs with single women."

- "I will only have affairs with women who my wife would not know."

- "I will only get on the computer after hours at work."

Eventually, the addict comes to break all of his own rules as he takes more and more risks. He starts to have affairs with women in his town, then a neighbor, and then a woman at his church. He starts to visit massage parlors in his own city and starts his day at work by downloading pornography.

When he continues his risky behavior despite negative consequences and he requires more and more to obtain the same effect, then addiction has set in, no matter what the specific behavior. The behavior will continue to progress and it will ultimately destroy the addict's life unless the cycle is disrupted with a new start in recovery.

Unlike complete abstinence that defines alcohol and drug recovery, sex addiction recovery does not require total abstinence from sex. In this way it is similar to recovery from compulsive overeating. Sexuality is a part of one's natural human state, as is the need to fuel one's body with food. People in recovery from eating disorders, specifically compulsive overeating, avoid eating certain foods. They learn to eat for the nutritional value of the food rather than eating out of boredom or to anesthetize anger or pain or other feelings. Ultimately, they develop a whole new relationship with the role of food in their life. In recovery, the sex addict also develops a whole new relationship with the role sex plays in his life. There will be certain behaviors he will no longer engage in. The act of sex will be for the experience, for the sharing of sexual pleasure, and for relational connection rather than out of his emotional reactivity and woundedness or for the sake of garnering power and control. He'll learn how to identify and voice his needs and feelings and to honor those of others, creating greater emotional and sexual intimacy. The recovering sex addict will develop boundaries that are based on respect for self and others. Whether the addiction is food, gambling, substances, or sex, all addicts in recovery learn how to identify their triggers and how to avoid them or not react in self-defeating ways. While all addicts need to develop greater emotional and relational skills to create healthier ways of getting their personal and interpersonal needs met, recovery for the sex addict is about learning how to get those needs met in a nonsexual way and addressing the issues that created barriers to healthy intimacy.

Why Am I Not Enough?

It is my hope that in better understanding the addictive nature of sexual compulsivity you will be able to answer the age-old question: *Why am I not enough?* Wives and partners often wonder why sex with them, and only them, is not sufficient for the sex addict. It's important to know that when the addict is in the throes of his addiction, he doesn't have sex with you to forge a connection and develop intimacy. He's doing it with you to keep up his pretenses, to reinforce your falsely held and unspoken belief that if he has sex with you then he isn't seeking it outside of your coupleship. Or you may simply be an element of his stash and part of his addictive cycle. In the act of his addiction—in the immediate moment—he may feel complete, whole, and good. But that feeling disappears once the activity is over, and he will go out and seek that feeling, as fleeting as it is, again and again.

[ADDICT]

I like having sex with my partner. She participates willingly and I find her attractive. I know she tries hard to please me. So why isn't that enough for me? All I can say is that my addiction isn't just about sex. There is this self-hate part of me that I try so hard to never show my wife. But when that self-hate gets triggered, and it is always there waiting to be triggered, that is when I act out. I have sex with women I don't know so I don't worry about displeasing them, nor do I have to be respectful to their needs. I also engage in totally different sexual acts that I would never ask my wife to engage in. My twisted thoughts about power, pain, and anger all come into play during my acting out. I am just into me, me, me, totally me.

The addict's feelings of shame, fear, and inadequacies are a bottomless pit. His behavior is an endless vicious cycle that has nothing to do with you.

Multiple Manifestations of Addiction

Addicted people often have histories of trauma, and the more profoundly they have been abused, the more likely they will have multiple addictive disorders. Some people have several forms of addiction operating simultaneously, while others trade off these forms (i.e., substances or behaviors), giving up one only to get lost in another. It is common that when one addiction is addressed, other addictive behaviors that do not get addressed gain strength. Many women have partners in recovery from one manifestation of addiction, such as alcohol, only to ultimately be confronted by sex addiction.

[ADDICT]

I got help for my alcoholism and I quit drinking because it was messing up everything. But I didn't give up all of my womanizing and affairs for another twenty years. I didn't see the sex messing up things. My marriage was struggling, but I just thought that was a problem between the two of us and had nothing to do with this secret world I had going on.

[ADDICT]

I used sex just as I used alcohol: to ignore pain, to block out my feelings. It separated me from a lot of loneliness, confusion, anger, guilt, and shame. I know I look like I have my act together to the outside world, but for my whole life, starting as a kid, I have felt lonely. I was never confident of myself. I was confused about why I did a lot of the things I did, and I felt guilty and ashamed. I sort of lived in two worlds: what I felt inside and what the world would see. They were two very different things. But I got good at buying into the outside image and ignoring that inner world. Well, that is exactly what alcohol and then sex did for me. They allowed me to disconnect from that inner world and believe my own lies about myself. I told myself that my behavior wasn't different from other men's behavior and that my behavior didn't really hurt anyone else because they didn't know about it.

Addicts will often seek help for the addiction that is most visible to others, the one they have the least shame about or the one that is the most disruptive to their lives. Addiction to substances, for example, are usually much more disruptive on a daily basis and are often more visible to others than sex addiction. It is also common for someone addicted to alcohol or other drugs or gambling to initially be willing to get help but continue to hold on to sexual secrets. Sometimes, while receiving help for one compulsive behavior, an addict is acting out in another addictive disorder because he believes he can handle it or thinks once he no longer uses drugs or drinks it will no longer be a problem. The denial and rationalizations about the hidden behavior go unrecognized. He does not fully understand that addiction takes on a life of its own. Unfortunately, many who get help for their identified addiction do not undergo any additional assessment for other problems. It's possible for his sexual acting out to continue for years before a crisis compels him to address his long-standing sexual compulsivity.

[ADDICT]

After ten years of being clean and sober from alcoholism, I knew I needed help again. I was not drinking or using. I was still going to a twelve-step program, but I was sexually acting out and being dishonest about our family money. Knowing it was catching up with me, and that my wife was very suspicious, I went to a treatment program. I had been to treatment ten years before, but I didn't get honest about anything but the alcohol. This time I told them I was in trouble for these other things.

The first time in treatment I thought that because my sexual acting out was always associated with my drinking that I just wouldn't do it if I didn't drink. And I also knew that if I exposed my sexual acting-out behaviors, they would want me to tell my wife, and I didn't want to do that. For two years I did okay, mostly because I just deliberately kept myself away from women as much as possible. But slowly I got myself back into my old behaviors. I was crazy in a sense because I knew what I was doing and knew I wasn't being honest with my recovery friends, my sponsor, or my wife. I was increasingly out of control. Shortly after my tenth sober anniversary

I got help for my sexual acting out because I also knew I was close to drinking again.

Addiction exists in layers. Some are more deeply embedded than others. Sometimes the various forms of addiction are ritualized together such as sex and alcohol or sex and other drugs (a form of speed such as cocaine or crystal methamphetamine is the most common). For example, an addict's ritual could be using crystal methamphetamine or cocaine as a part of his pattern of sexual acting out. Combining speed with sex is a way that addicts try to find an even greater high. After acting out, an addict will often use alcohol or marijuana to induce a greater sense of calmness in coming down from the previous high. Typically, this means that a person does not engage with one addictive behavior without engaging in another addictive behavior.

Work, rage, drugs, alcohol, sex, spending, gambling—it doesn't matter what the behavior or substance is, if it has the ability to (falsely) empower, to medicate or soothe, to help you avoid, and/or to move you from a feeling of "less than" to "better than," then it can be addictive. A man in recovery from addiction told me, "I was an addiction binger and trader."

[ADDICT]

I started a paper route when I was just a kid and found that work was a source of pride and solace. It got me out of the house and distracted me from all my fears. The money I made gave me independence. I became quite the entrepreneur and soon had other kids working for me. Reading was another source of solace and a way for me to disconnect from the pain and confusion of my life. I was really very angry with my father during that time, and my paper route and withdrawing into reading and numbers (I loved overseeing my bank account) gave me a sense of well-being and confidence that ultimately fueled a strong work and gambling addiction. Then I began to drink, and it too gave me a sense of well-being. Adding sex to that made it become one big, powerful cocktail.

Problems and behaviors that are often overlooked include raging behaviors, compulsive spending, and work obsession. Work obsession and distorted thinking about money are culturally supported, and rageful behavior is often hidden and a last vestige of recovery.

[ADDICT]

Rage, alcohol, marijuana, work, and sex—all were my validation. They also became my form of power. After I got sober, my sexual behavior went underground and my rage became sporadic, but my work addiction flared. I was on a seesaw, professing recovery. Finally I decided to do some therapy around my childhood. It was then that a clinician confronted me about my sexual behavior. This led to my issues with rage and work addiction being addressed in my recovery.

Another prevalent combination of addictive behaviors is violence, drugs/alcohol, and sex. The violence component nearly always has its roots in a childhood that included parents or caregivers who were alcoholic, physically violent, and/or sexually abusive. In some cases, the child received affection only after being abused or after a family fight. Thus, for that person, violence and affection (sex) are paired. It may be that as a young boy the addict listened to his parents arguing and heard the physical abuse as his father literally threw his mother around the bedroom. In his powerlessness as a young child, he found comfort in masturbation. Today he cannot get an erection unless he fantasizes about something of a violent nature while listening to music with violent lyrics. When addiction is ritualized, each manifestation feeds the other and intensifies the addictive cycle.

To keep from merely switching addictions and to support a healthy recovery, the addict must identify and address all his forms of addictions as well as the internal source of his pain. Today, addiction specialists recognize that having multiple forms of addiction is interactive; they present as a package. If you cut off or treat just one branch of a diseased tree, it does not necessarily heal or get to the root of the problem. Whether there are dual or multiple forms of addiction, each manifestation is a primary issue, and each needs to be addressed simultaneously.

Even though not all sex addicts are addicted to alcohol and other drugs, all reputable sexual addiction treatment programs strongly advise abstinence from alcohol and any so-called recreational drug use since any use is a disinhibiter. These substances weaken a person's judgment to the point that one cannot remain committed to healthy boundaries, which are a part of recovery from sex addiction. They can strongly influence a relapse into addictive thinking, which sets up the addictive behavior.

Any process or behavior that interferes with the ability to be honest deserves attention—whether it is addiction or an otherwise, self-defeating behavior that doesn't support healing and recovery.

Depression and Anxiety

It is common for addicts to experience underlying depression and anxiety as a consequence of both biology and traumatic family histories. In addition to a generalized anxiety disorder, post-traumatic stress often underlies addiction. These co-occurring mental health disorders may be substance-related but very often are their own primary issue. Like multiple manifestations of addiction, depression and anxiety often go unrecognized for many years. It is not uncommon for a sex addict to seek treatment for substance abuse, then ultimately for his sex addiction, and then without a substance or behavior to give him false esteem or to medicate, his underlying depression and anxiety become much more apparent. While we all know the typical symptoms of depression are apathy, lethargy, and feeling blue, it is not uncommon, particularly for men, for depression to be expressed as blatant hostility and unmanageable anger and rage. The symptoms of undiagnosed disorders such as depression and anxiety can be masked and managed through patterns of addictive and compulsive behavior.

[ADDICT]

I am not the kind of guy who thinks of himself as depressed, but in my recovery from sex addiction I was still acting out with explosive anger and really rageful behavior. My size, words, and loudness are intimidating, and I used them. A therapist suggested antidepressants, and I had learned to be open to suggestions from those I respected. To be honest, I was shocked by the recommendation, but now it is apparent that alcohol and sex just covered up this depression. My anger was always close by, always ready to protect me. So depression was just more and more apparent without my other fixes. Today I still have some inappropriate anger, but that is not so related to depression as just a lifetime of being quick to use anger, and it's my first defense. But treating my depression has made a world of difference that I never would have identified as an issue for me. After all, big men are not supposed to be depressed.

Addictive behavior—whether it's satiation, arousal, or fantasy—can be a cover to depression. In our society, it is far more acceptable for a man to get treatment for addiction than to be diagnosed with and treated for depression. It is considered unmanly to be depressed. In our culture, girls and women are socialized to internalize pain; they blame themselves and draw distress into themselves. Boys and men are socialized to externalize pain and are more likely to discharge distress through action. A man is running from the pain and emptiness he has felt for years, engaging compulsively in work, financial goals, and sex. Money, prowess, and prestige become the drugs that sustain him and take the place of authentic relationships. He has trouble being intimate with others because he can't be intimate with himself. His sexual acting out is an attempt to escape the sense of unworthiness and emotional impoverishment that has haunted him throughout much of his life. To relieve the threat of depression, the addictive substance or process in this case works to transform the emotional state from feelings of worthlessness to feelings of extraordinary worth.

As Terrence Real so eloquently says in *I Don't Want To Talk About It*, "the depressed man frequently buries himself in work, wraps his internal discomfort in anger, and numbs his discontent with alcohol, other drugs, and sex. As a society we have more respect for the walking wounded, those who persist, deny their pain and difficulties."[5] Men readily engage in satiating and fantasy behavior, and at the same time they are pushed toward arousal-type behaviors. They are expected to engage in risk-taking but are to avoid being vulnerable or owning or showing those feelings. Pain is something they are to rise above. As a consequence, an addict's untreated depression sabotages his recovery.

[ADDICT]

I went to AA because my wife threatened to leave me due to my drinking. She knew about some of my sexual acting out but thought it only happened because of my drinking. The truth was I drank more in response to the shame I felt about my acting out. But who really knew that? So I went to AA to save my marriage. I was also tired of all the drinking and I couldn't seem to stop. But when I went to AA, I left half of me outside the door. Then in time, with recovery from alcoholism, I found food to be the solace that alcohol once was to hide my sexual shame. So I had this odd fight going on of esteem building in AA, yet I had this secretive sex life. Finally my growing esteem took me to Overeaters Anonymous (OA). Now where were my fixes? I couldn't hide from myself, and my sexual acting out was leaking everywhere. My dishonesty was challenged by the principles of the twelve-step programs. That was when I finally got help for my sex addiction, and soon after I was in full-blown depression.

Current research confirms that a vulnerability to depression is genetically inherited. Any person, given the right mix of chromosomes, will have a susceptibility to this disease. Major depression and bipolar disorder are the two forms of depression most likely linked to biology—a genetic history. Bipolar disorder is characterized not only by depressive symptoms, but by a switching between what are referred to as the poles of manic and depressive episodes. These episodes can vary in duration and intensity, depending on the person. Bipolar disorder has a specific link to sex addiction because one of the symptoms of bipolar disorder can be hypersexuality. *Hypersexuality* is the increased need, even pressure, for sexual gratification driven in part by the physical activation, heightened sensory and sexual interest, and risk-taking that are often symptoms of mania for a person with bipolar disorder. With the exception of bipolar disorder, in the majority of cases, biological vulnerability alone is not enough to bring about depression. Usually a combination of genetic susceptibility and psychological injury produces depression. Such psychological injury—especially physical or sexual abuse or being raised in extremely impaired family systems—is often seen in men who act out sexually. Many times the dominating source of impairment in his family was an addiction that created loss and modeled addictive behavior as a solution to pain or a source of power.

It is also possible the addict may experience *dysthymia* (low-grade, chronic depression) due to the shame he feels as he confronts his behavior and the sense of emptiness or hollowness that often accompanies the initial absence of his acting out. When diagnosed appropriately, depression of all types can be treated quite effectively with medication and/or psychotherapy. As with addiction, a strong diagnostic work-up in a treatment process is advisable to identify or rule out mental health issues that could interfere with and/ or sabotage the recovery process. The most common issues are depression, anxiety, and post-traumatic stress symptoms, most often due to childhood abuse. This may seem overwhelming, but neither you nor your partner need to carve the path of treatment, as a qualified sex addiction therapist will do this. With a desire and willingness to change, recovery is possible.

If you see a repetitive pattern to your partner's behavior, and if he continues his behaviors in spite of adverse consequences to himself, to you, and to his family, it is most likely this behavior needs to be addressed with a specific addiction focus and not just seen as a painful lapse in relationship fidelity or an innate perversion. There are emotional reasons for this acting out that ultimately lead to repetition and compulsivity, and the inability to willfully control himself. Of course, these explanations don't excuse his behavior; what they do is contribute to understanding. It is also important to know that there is a path for treatment and healing.

Reflective Thoughts and Questions

- What did you learn in this chapter that helps you understand your partner's behavior?

- In what way does understanding the addictive nature of his behavior aid you in your recovery?

- Are you concerned about your partner having other addictions? Explain.

- Are you concerned that he may have depression, anxiety, and/or other mental health issues? Explain.

- What was important for you to learn in this chapter?

CHAPTER THREE NOTES

1   Benjamin Franklin, *The Autobiography of Benjamin Franklin* (New York: Touchstone, 2003), 55.

2   Wilt Chamberlain, *A View from Above* (New York: Signet, 1992).

3   Harvey Milkman and Stanley Sunderwirth, *Craving for Ecstacy: How Our Passions Become Addictions and What We Can Do About Them* (San Francisco: Jossey-Bass, 1987).

4   Patrick Carnes, *Contrary to Love: Helping the Sexual Addict* (Center City, MN: Hazelden, 1994).

5   Terrence Real, *I Don't Want to Talk about It: Overcoming the Secret Legacy of Male Depression* (New York: Simon & Schuster, 1998), 35.

CHAPTER FOUR

Generational Repeat

Why does this feel so familiar?

What familial traits do my partner and I have in common?

For many partners, it is not coincidental that you are in a relationship with an addict. It may feel very familiar; however, you don't deserve to be treated with disrespect.

In some sectors of our culture, socialization of women sets them up to defer to men by giving them the benefit of the doubt, taking on false guilt, believing they need a man to have value, and prioritizing his needs over their own. Women are taught to acquiesce, be polite, and refrain from showing anger. They often feel inadequate about their sexuality or have a distorted and shame-based body image. This conditions a woman to be easily manipulated and gaslighted leading her to victimization and consequently reinforces the trauma of sexual betrayal.

Yet your family history could be more influential than the cultural socialization While you may not have thought of your childhood as being significant to what is happening now, and while there is no such thing as perfect parenting or perfect families, looking at family history and dynamics will be significant in your healing. It's critical to examine the beliefs you developed about yourself and others, the ways you learned to experience connection and/or protect yourself, and the behaviors that helped you to garner esteem.

The behaviors and belief systems of both partners and sex addicts are strongly influenced by individual childhood experiences. It is common that one or both parents suffered with addiction, most commonly alcohol and/or other drugs or sexual addiction. While this "affliction/malady" may not have been called addiction, their father was known as a womanizer or their mother had a lot of affairs or drank a lot, and so on. If not addiction, there were often other forms of family impairment or dysfunction that would create wounds that led to addiction and unhealthy ways of coping in relationships. There may have been a history of extreme parental rigidity, strict all-or-nothing parental codes. Messages about sex were distorted or shaming, therefore creating confusion and pain for their children.

More often than not, both members of the coupleship were raised in family systems in which they experienced a range of emotional and physical abandonment.

Abandonment

Physical abandonment means that a person's basic physical needs are not attended to consistently. A child looks to his parent for food, shelter, clothing, and appropriate supervision. Any time a child experiences physical and/or sexual abuse that is considered physical abandonment. If you were not afforded the protection, the safety, and the security you needed to thrive, you experienced abandonment.

When you feel that you have to hide major aspects of your being in order to be accepted or to protect yourself, this is abandonment. When you believe it is not physically or psychologically safe to make a mistake, to have your own needs, to have accomplishments, or to freely express the range of feelings that are part of the human experience, this is abandonment. If boundaries were lacking, permissive, too rigid, or otherwise seriously distorted, if you were expected to live out another person's dreams or to engage in peer-like relationships with those in the parental role, or if your parents' expectations were not age-appropriate, then you have experienced abandonment.

Physical or emotional abandonment is hurtful, painful, and traumatic to a child's development. Depending on the severity of abandonment, it can be disruptive to healthy self-esteem, your sense of worth and value, emotional maturity, and social and relational skills. In psychological terms this is regarded as *arrested development*. As a result of abandonment, what you see is that both of you can act out in similar, and at the same time very different ways.

THE PARTNER: TRAUMA REPETITION

Kate has much in common with the other women sharing their stories in this book. She was raised in an alcoholic and violent family. She is divorced from two different alcoholic men and is now married to an active sex addict. Her husband has had multiple relationships with other women and now he is flagrantly acting out in a manner that she cannot totally deny. She knows he sees prostitutes and on a recent visit to one, he brought their four-year-old son with him. Yet she still has the ability to rationalize: "He is stressed by our two young children. He wouldn't do this if he weren't on drugs." She deliberately does not ask questions. If she doesn't ask, then it is as if she doesn't have to know. She doesn't ask for help because, as she says, "I just need him to stop." She doesn't assert any limits because her fear is that he will leave her. In ultimate desperation she finds herself left alone in a hotel room with a baby just a few weeks old and a four-year-old, no car, no food, and no money while he goes to get more drugs and meet up with a girlfriend; and she just wants him back.

Kate didn't get to this place overnight. Her childhood history was her training ground long before she entered any of her three addictive relationships. As with most partners of addicts, dysfunction ruled her original family. As a child, she learned to:

- Overlook (deny, rationalize, minimize) behavior that hurt her deeply

- Appear cheerful when she is hurting

- Make excuses for the hurtful behavior

- Avoid conflict to minimize further anger

- Tolerate inappropriate and hurtful behavior

- Prioritize the needs of others over her own needs

- Take care of others

- Fault herself for her family's problems

- Discount her own perceptions, giving others the benefit of the doubt

- Believe she has no options available

- Not ask for help

- Accommodate

Kate was reared to be the perfect candidate for partnering with an addict. A natural consequence of being raised in a shame-based family, very often an abusive or addictive family, is that the child grows up to be an ideal partner for an addict, one whose trauma and childhood survivor traits enable him to act out his addiction with little disruption.

[ADDICT]

I look back now and know that my wife was the perfect partner for me to be able to have this other life. She always wanted to believe me. I controlled her with anger. She had been raised by a raging father, and then her stepfather sexually abused her. All I had to do was raise my voice and ask, "How can you doubt me after all I do for you? You should be grateful." I'd see the shift in her eyes and she would crumble. Then I'd switch to telling her everything was okay, telling her I really loved her, and acting like I forgave her for her suspicions.

As each manifestation of Kate's husbands' addiction escalated her fears of abandonment and rejection also escalated driving her to engage in maladaptive behaviors. She became more compulsive in her busyness, which wasn't hard with two young children and a part-time job. If she kept busy enough, she didn't have to feel or see. If she was good enough, no one could find fault with her, nor would her current husband ever want to leave her. The busier she got, the more depressed and anxious she became. Her esteem eroded; her neediness surged. Each marriage ended with her husband leaving. Their addiction became so severe they could not shoulder any responsibility. The divorces simply reinforced Kate's feeling that she was flawed in some fundamental way.

While the names change, the stories of repetitively partnering with an addict are common and span generations. What Kate and other partners often experience is referred to as *trauma repetition.* Although Kate repeated it many times in her own life, others repeat it generationally. When you find yourself in the same situation with the same type of person over and over again, you seldom link the behavior to your original betrayal and trauma. Reenactment is living in the irreconcilable past. You may have been raised with addiction in your household and may even have that knowledge, but that doesn't necessarily keep you from marrying addictive and/or abusive men. Replaying your past trauma is often repeating what you know, the familiar, or what you believe you deserve. Patrick Carnes, in *The Betrayal Bond,* summarizes trauma repetition as characterized "by 1) doing something self-destructive over and over again, usually something that took place in childhood and started with a trauma; 2) reliving a 'story' from the past; 3) engaging in abusive relationships repeatedly; 4) repeating painful experiences, including specific behaviors, scenes, persons and feelings."[1] Ultimately, it is as futile as attempting to survive the sinking *Titanic* by repeatedly changing your seat as the ship is going down.

Sara also has a history of repetitively changing alcoholic and/or sex-addicted partners, repeating her generational family patterns. Yet by recognizing her trauma repetition, by claiming her inner voice and embracing acts of recovery, she let go of her role of family savior and moved on with the business of changing her life.

[SARA]

My life has been riddled with the horror trauma. My father committed suicide when I was only a year old. My mother had just left him due to his "womanizing" (that's what they called it back then). Today we know it as sex addiction. My Irish family was filled with alcoholics and sex addicts. I stayed with my aunts until my mother remarried when I was five. I began believing early on that if I could just keep the peace, protect my cousins, stop the depression, everyone would be happy, and then I would be safe. This illusion of control grew throughout my life, and I would repeat my family's history over and over. My idea of an attractive man was my uncle, a hard drinking, raging, handsome woman-chaser. Over the years I realized I didn't have a chance. I was attracted to the image burned into my little psyche long ago. Over and over, unconsciously, I would try to solve the problem, fix history, and create a new ending. I just added a new twist: change the ending by just being better, explaining the hurt effectively, and magically transforming the outcome for our families and us.

Like other Women of the Lodge, the following partner readily identifies with the analogy of changing seats on the *Titanic* as it is sinking. She found that by recognizing a need to "fill herself up from the inside with greater esteem and skills" that there was a lifeboat available to her.

[PARTNER]

My boyfriend and I broke up after a few years of his acting out. He was never willing to get help. I spent those years trying to be the person I thought he needed or wanted me to be. I did a lot of things that I regret today. When I left, I simply wanted out—I was running. Then I ran right into another one of him. He looked different on the outside, but within a few months I found out I was just one of his harem. Funny how things happen, but I was seeing things in magazines, on talk shows, and on other television shows about women who repeat their relationships time after time with different guys. I know I had heard this before, but somehow I heard it differently. I guess I was ready. So I threw myself into lots of self-help reading. You would have thought the authors knew me firsthand. It helped me not feel so stupid. I knew I wasn't alone. I have a lot of girlfriends like me. But I thought all this time it was the guys who were bad and we were just stupid. Well, I am not stupid. I have made mistakes but I have come to realize I didn't know how to do it differently, and I had a lot I could work on that would lead me in a different path. So I set about learning how to trust myself. Figuring out what made me feel good in life. I developed my own interests so I wasn't just attaching myself to someone else. To do this I had to be willing to *not* date. That actually was a relief. And then one day I realized I wasn't going to hang on to my resentments, I didn't need them; my life wasn't about these guys, it was about me. Funny how once I took the focus off them, suddenly I knew in my heart they weren't bad guys. They maybe did or didn't love me along the way, but they didn't know how to love me or how to do it in a healthy way. I found forgiveness for me and for them. But that doesn't mean I have to live with or marry them.

Perhaps you have entered into a relationship with someone who has the same addiction as your parent, but because you were so young when your parent was in the early stages of addiction you have no distinct recall of it. People often don't realize there are early, middle, and late stages to addictive disorders. Because of this, women often don't see the similarities between a partner's addiction and a parent's addiction because they were in different stages. Or maybe, like many women, you are so focused on making sure you don't end up with a partner like your alcoholic or drug-addicted father, that you are ever vigilant to look for someone who appears to drink responsibly or who doesn't drink or use drugs at all, that you end up ignoring the signs of other addictive behavior.

[PARTNER]

My father was a raging alcoholic. No one in my family ever spoke up to him; we lived in fear of speaking up, and yet when he handed out favors,

I was his favorite. I was hungry for his attention, hungry for his approval. And it was the setup for a perfect match for the sex addict, really any kind of addict. But I was so busy making sure it was not someone who looked out of control, like my father with his drinking and rage, so I was looking for the "class president" and in doing so, not realizing I was simply a magnet for another kind of addiction. I was the perfect match for the high-achieving, professionally visible sex addict. For over thirty-four years I was obsessed with my husband's behavior. My whole existence was in attempting to know the details of where he was, when, and with whom. In that time I managed to raise three children, and today my middle daughter is repeating my marriage exactly. I shouldn't be surprised at this, as I had repeated my mother's marriage, with a slight variation, and as I look at my family history, I see that she repeated her mother's marriage.

This repetition has long been recognized as expressed in the following quote: "The gods visit the sins of the fathers upon the children."[2]

[VANESSA]

Much of my recovery work has taken me back to my childhood. I have had to repeatedly work through the core belief that I am not good enough. I was the reason my parents got married; they had to—a sad beginning for an unwanted baby entering a loveless marriage. To compound the situation, I was supposed to be a boy to take over the family business. I carried an anti-female stigma with me most of my life. Even my gender wasn't good enough. Both of my parents were work addicts. My dad was rarely home, leaving before I woke up and home long after I went to bed. When he was home, either he was raging and belittling my sister and me or eerily quiet. My mother seemed to have little time for nurturing. On the outside we were a typical religious family and strictly admonished to ensure the world believed that. Clearly we operated with the theme: Don't talk. Don't talk about any problems or feelings you might have. If you can't say anything nice, don't say it at all. Do what you're told. And most important, never talk outside of home. We didn't air our dirty laundry, whatever it was. Combine that with the idea that we were only to show good feelings, which of course meant to suppress anything that wasn't a happy face. Don't feel. My sister and I were highly disciplined, smiling, perfect little girls. I took that discipline into my adult life and became a party girl/work addict. And who would I choose for a partner? Not a rager, not a workaholic, but another type of addict.

Perhaps you are aware of your partner's behavior but have minimal expectations due to low self-esteem wherein you don't expect more out of life. You see yourself as a survivor; you believe you can tolerate and handle things.

[PARTNER]

I've had two husbands who left me after years of my putting up with both of them having multiple affairs, from one-night stands to longstanding girlfriends. It never dawned on me to leave or that I could confront them or ask for anything different. I felt so poorly about myself. I allowed myself to be degraded and belittled, all the while projecting this false bravado of being tough. I acted like a victim-martyr, and all it did was fuel my depression.

Dysfunction in families occurs along a continuum. You do not have to be raised with addiction to partner with addiction as an adult. Abuse, addiction, and mental illness are blatant sources of dysfunction; their common denominator is loss—loss of nurturing and safety. Within other types of families, loss certainly exists but is more subtle, such as in families where the parenting and relational styles are rigid or too permissive. Families that are highly enmeshed and those with severe relational disconnection also fuel similar behaviors. Many women strongly believe they were raised in healthy families, but as they explore their behaviors they come to recognize how aspects of their growing-up years may be impacting their coping strategies today. This is not about blame but about recognizing generational influences that will help you focus on your recovery needs.

[PARTNER]

My being so powerless in my marriage came from a long history of being powerless. I was raised with two older brothers and I was the baby. I had a very emotionally neglectful home. It looked good on the outside, and my parents looked loving, available, and responsible. However, in reality, they were emotionally absent and emotionally neglectful. They never taught me about the outside world. I was sheltered from reality, very naïve, and sexually shamed. What I mean by this is that it was immature or shameful to have normal romantic longing. As an adolescent, I remember them making fun of my friends who had crushes on boys or who had pictures of male celebrities on their bedroom walls. Or if a couple was being affectionate in public they would say something like "Look at those two, they ought to be ashamed of themselves!" or "Don't they know better?" or "They must have been raised in a barn." The implication was that no civilized, educated person had romantic or sexual longings. I never saw affection or any sexual energy between my parents. The only thing they would show was a bird peck kiss on the lips as my dad would leave for work. I remember thinking it looked strained and like neither one of them really enjoyed it, but it was the thing to do. So I learned from this that sex was bad and that it was only to have children. I learned to be ashamed of and afraid of my own longings for intimacy and sexuality. I felt like I was always on stage with my parents, and I learned to act like I was on stage with everyone that I knew.

Prior to her marriage, this woman had already internalized an overwhelming sense of helplessness, a sense of defeat. She had also learned the art of *image management*—how not to be real or authentic but to be "on stage" and in character. The negative messages she inherited about sex and sexuality set her up for confusion and self-doubt about healthy sexuality and poor sexual esteem in her marriage. Coupled with her overall low self-esteem, she was easily exploited by her sexually compulsive husband.

Therese, like the previous woman, was raised in a family who failed to acknowledge her sexuality or curiosity. She internalized sexual shame because she didn't learn healthy expressions of sexuality or acknowledgment of it. "It was shameful to have romantic longings. Affection was perceived as disgusting." Image was also very important in her household, which meant she had no opportunity to learn how to deal with conflict, times of fear, and uncertainty.

[THERESE]

My friends thought my family was the best and always wanted to be at my house. Our house was safe and full of good feelings; only good feelings. What a distortion of reality. Anything that was contrary to good feelings only had a short life before it was ousted or pushed underground, never to be acknowledged again. There was total dismissal of the struggles a girl could have as a teenager and I couldn't be anything but fine or great. Anything else just didn't go with the image.

When my husband first acted out, I felt like I couldn't tell anyone. Who would I tell? I was so ashamed. I couldn't risk breaking the image that everyone had of me and our marriage. I was so emotionally isolated that I didn't tell my closest and only girlfriend. I kept it buried inside of me. I felt like my husband's need for pornography and other women implied that I was not good enough for him. To compensate and cope with my growing feelings of unworthiness, I lost track of myself and became what anyone else wanted. I began to drown in my worry, fear, and shame.

Like many, Therese grew up in a family that taught her that only good feelings were acceptable. She got the message that she was to defer to others and give them the benefit of the doubt over herself—that other people's needs were more important than hers. In her family she did not learn conflict resolution skills, therefore had little modeling for healthy communication, and because the focus was on image or outcome, she didn't learn about being intimate and chose a partner with similar traits.

Couple that with any history of family abandonment, it's often easier to deny and/or tolerate the painful reality of being in an actively addicted relationship than to not, which for so many women tap into your feeling of abandonment. That feeling of abandonment then translates into the pain that comes with the belief that you are not worthy, not of value. Whatever the influences, this is the time not to be judgmental but to empathize with yourself. But it is important to look at any family history that fuels your traumatic stress and your traumatic responses. Ultimately, without recovery from childhood wounding, you won't have the foundation to maintain new recovery skills. There is a path from which you can let go of your self-defeating thoughts and behaviors. You can actualize a stronger sense of self based on esteem. But it means you have to act, not react.

SEXUAL MESSAGES

Partners and the sex addict have both frequently received unhealthy messages about sexuality when they were children. It is common for one or the other of them to have experienced sexual abuse. Some experienced overt, blatant incest or molestation. It is from this experience that children can come to believe that sex is what you do to be lovable or to gain attention, or it's the only way they know to experience power or control and avoid victimization. The abuse can also fuel conflicting feelings, ranging from guilt and shame to fear and excitement about sexuality.

The sexual abuse may have been more covert or subtle. Some children were never touched inappropriately themselves, but they may have witnessed adult sexual activities or were subjected to repeated comments about their bodies or their sexual development or were exposed to pornography. Home may have been a highly charged sexual atmosphere with sexually explicit jokes, sexualized clothing, or frequent sexual innuendos. A sexually restricted family where children are taught that sex is bad, dirty, or disgusting is unhealthy as well. These children don't know what healthy sexuality is. Families where sexual boundaries are distorted or nonexistent are a breeding ground for people who will eventually act out sexually and those who will partner with them. In these situations, children are abandoned and violated, and they learn how to deny pain.

[PARTNER]

My stepfather sexually abused me for several years. I didn't tell anyone. By the time I was a teenager, I was proud of my ability to get any guy into bed. I just wanted their attention, and I felt that was the way to get it. To me, it meant being noticed, not discarded. In time it became my source of power. I got this warped sense of esteem from my promiscuity. I have had to grapple with my own sexual compulsivity as I have had to grapple the issues of sexual betrayal. Because I have had so much shame around my own previous behavior, it has been hard for me to think I was worthy of asking for more in a relationship. But I am learning I deserve more than abuse and addiction in my life.

[JACQUE]

I was abused by my older brother for several years when I was only a small child. He would come into my bedroom late at night and literally threaten my life, sometimes with a knife, if I didn't do what he wanted. I was a sex toy for him. By late adolescence, I felt so degraded and worthless I set out to prove I was of value. I'd go to bars, flirt, drink, and see how many guys I could attract. It was a vicious cycle because in the moment I would feel invincible yet it ultimately only eroded what little esteem I had. In many ways, by participating in my husband's sexual fantasies I was repeating my cycle of thinking it made me desirable to him, yet feeling humiliated for myself. I was now an adult allowing myself to be victimized. I have struggled a lot with signs of posttraumatic stress, particularly with an inability to manage my emotions. My fear and anxiety only fueled greater victimization because I was too frightened to set boundaries and didn't think I was worthy of having them. I'd often use alcohol to numb myself. My recovery as a sexual abuse survivor actually began prior to my knowing that I was dealing with sex addiction.

[JENNY]

I know now that I had been objectified as a child by my dad. There was no overt sexual abuse by him but there was covert sexualization just by the feelings that I got when I would wear a dress. I didn't like those feelings so I continued to want to be a boy. By being a tomboy I could get my dad's attention and affection, but as a "pretty girl" I felt that he was uncomfortable with me. At about age twelve I discovered some pornography in my parents' bedroom. I remember feeling afraid and somehow dirty. I think of my family life as abusive from the standpoint that it was sexually neglectful. No one ever talked about sex, and it was taboo.

The only education I even got about my own body and reproductive system was at school in the sixth grade, and I was so ashamed during the class that I couldn't really listen or learn. Everything about my body—sexual feelings, romantic desires, and even menstruation—was shameful and had to be denied at any cost. I believe these things are a part of my history that set me up to tolerate my partner's sexual acting out and to be abused sexually by him.

When the only way you are validated by a significant other who is supposed to love you is through sex, you can develop a twisted belief that sex is love. It can set you up for your own sexual acting out and/or be the reason that you are attracted to a man who acts out sexually, allowing you to be exploited by him. Jacque, who was sexually abused by her brother for four to six years while growing up, resumed her role as a sexual victim in her adult life. She agreed to participate in some of her husband's addictive behavior such as performing sexually at a club. She struggled with honoring herself and her desire not to participate, but she craved validation from her husband. Many women feel ashamed about what they have willingly engaged in sexually to placate a partner. Women such as Jenny struggle with any sense of what feels good to them sexually, as sex is not okay—it is simply an act they engage in, hoping for love.

To grow up with addiction and/or sexual abuse means you learned to distrust your own perceptions. As children share their thoughts with adults, they are frequently discounted and so they spend their entire lives doubting the truth of their own experiences and pretending they were never hurt. They stop trusting their own intuition or their own version of reality. That is as damaging as the violation itself and certainly is trauma in the making.

When both addiction and sex abuse occur during childhood, dysfunctional beliefs and needed defenses—such as not talking about your feelings, not trusting others, not asking for help, and so on—are doubly reinforced. For example, if you are raised in a situation where there is either addiction or abuse, you will have difficulty trusting others. But if you are raised in a situation where both occur, you will have even greater difficulty trusting others, as there is a synergistic effect. One plus one does not equal two; now it equals three. Those raised in households with either addiction or abuse will have a high tolerance for inappropriate behavior. Those raised in households with both addiction and abuse will have an even higher tolerance for inappropriate and hurtful behavior. Clearly, it is hurtful to be raised with addiction and/or abuse; when they coexist, the negative consequences reinforce each other.

Covert sexual abuse such as drunken nudity, sexual name-calling, or the lack of appropriate sexual information during childhood creates confusion regarding healthy sexuality; it aids in high tolerance for inappropriate behavior and may fuel shame around one's sexual feelings and behavior. Overt sexual abuse such as molestation is a much blatant betrayal and violation and a far greater emotional, physical, and spiritual injustice. A person with this experience is more likely to encounter any of the following and often a combination: to 1) dissociate (separating emotions from thoughts as if existing outside her physical being and controlling her actions by remote control); 2) regard sex as a form of control and power; 3) equate sex with love; 4) view sexuality as the primary source of his or her identity.

As the addict often has underlying and co-occurring problems of depression and anxiety, partners, those in particular who grew up in impaired family systems, also often enter the relationship with undiagnosed major depression or dysthymia (low-grade, chronic depression), anxiety, and/or post-traumatic stress. The likelihood that you entered your relationship with these issues is higher for you than others, if you were raised in a shame-based, addictive, and/or verbally, physically, or sexually abusive family system. If you entered your relationship with depression, low self-esteem, self-defeating thoughts, and/or shame-based defenses, it aids an environment in which the addict is safe to maintain his secret double life without being caught or held accountable. As discussed in Chapter Two, the more trauma you have had in your life, the greater the impact of traumatic stress when there is sexual betrayal in your adult relationship.

Your first efforts in understanding how your past is influencing your current behavior begins with exploring the dynamics in the family in which you were raised. For many, the roots of addiction may in fact span generations. It is essential to look back at your early life and identify the critical experiences that shaped you. This is the beginning of the road to your healing. Consider these questions:

- What words would you use to describe your family when you were growing up?

- What messages did you get about having needs? How has that been hurtful or helpful to you?

- Was it okay for you to express your opinions?

- What messages were you given about being female? How has that been hurtful or helpful to you?

- What messages were you given about being male? How has that been hurtful or helpful to you?

- What messages did you receive about being sexual? How has that been hurtful or helpful to you?

- How have those messages influenced your present-day situation?

- How would you describe the use of alcohol or other drugs in your family?

- Are you aware of any family history of physical or sexual abuse?

- What addictive or abusive behaviors are you aware of generationally?

- How do you think your family dynamic has contributed to your being in a relationship with an addict?

THE ADDICT: REENACTING THE WOUND

As recovering sex addicts review their histories, many recognize they come from strongly impaired family systems, families impacted by various addictive disorders and forms of mental illnesses. Situations of physical and sexual violence are extremely common. Often these boys had emotionally unavailable fathers and highly enmeshed relationships with their mothers. With their dysfunctional histories, these are emotionally wounded boys who learn to project to the world one persona but act out another.

Just as the partner often identifies with trauma repetition, so too does the addict. But the addict also perpetuates the affront to him. This means that in addition to reliving a story from the past, continuing to engage in self-destructive behaviors over and over again, and repeating painful experiences, addicts often do to others what they experienced as an early life trauma. Maureen Canning, author of *Lust, Anger, Love*, writes, "All sexual acting out is motivated by feelings of shame and manifested in acts and feelings of anger."[3] They are men (and women) who have become the perpetrators of their own pain and of the pain of others.

[ADDICT]

By the time I was thirteen I was so angry I wanted to scream, but I had no way to do that. What do you do with that anger when you're just a kid? I was angry about life in general—too many divorces by my parents, too many moves, total neglect by my father, and rage from my stepfather. My mom loved me but she was too caught up in her life to know how to cope with my problems at school or my depression. My first way to "scream" was by skipping school, and then I found porn on the internet. My hormones were starting to rage, sex became the answer to my pain and anger, and I was on my way.

In the movie *Prince of Tides*, the character played by Nick Nolte explains how when his parents began their war against each other the only prisoners they took were their children, and how the kids developed a ritual to escape—they found a silent soothing world of no pain. For many, this is what addiction is about: a silent soothing world, a world of no pain. A world of disconnection—kindled by fear and shame, often rooted in trauma.

[ADDICT]

At age eleven I had a hole in my gut that was so big only alcohol and drugs would fill it up. It would become my answer—my solution—and I would get blithering numb. Then I found masturbation and pornography, and they took me to another realm. For a moment all I knew was my escape from feeling unwanted and unloved. Now I needed no one. I had me.

[ADDICT]

Masturbation was a form of escape and solace when I was just a young boy. I'd often take myself to an open lot down the alley from our house and spend my time alone, fantasizing and masturbating. It was actually in that lot where I found my first pornography. The sexual pleasure of pornography and masturbating made a powerful tie when I was anxious, stressed, and scared. My mother was very domineering and volatile. She disciplined in anger, physically, with belts. Dad took the path of least resistance. He left us kids to take the explosion. He was very demanding, though, with high expectations. He pushed us hard in sports and academics. Because we were physically small, he pushed us even harder to be the best. I'd use masturbation to wake up in the morning, as an eye opener. It got me up and moving. It was a way for me to calm myself and to go to sleep when I was anxious. As I got older, I'd also use sex as a reward. I would tell myself I was entitled, that my behavior didn't hurt anyone else.

Pretty crazy thinking, but it had become a predominant source of reward, way to relax, and a boost of esteem. It quickly became my answer to fear. I was just this overgrown, scared, terrified little boy inside.

Strongly influenced by his childhood history, an addict uses his sexuality to meet different needs. Pleasurable feelings of sexuality were perhaps the only relief he ever knew during childhood. Sex was his escape, a mood-altering experience. As he grew up, sex continued to be a means of coping with stress. Early on, the addict learned to use fantasy and arousal to stabilize his mood temporarily or to avoid anxiety. Later, as he discovered sexual pleasure, fantasy served an even more powerful and distracting role, and the addict began to lose himself in it in a way that characterizes sexual acting out. When an addict begins to feel something painful, he uses sex as a way to medicate that pain. Even fantasizing without personal physical contact can be soothing to a sex addict.

When stressed by any difficult situation (whether it is work, family, money, or loneliness), addicts turn to using an external substance or engaging in an addictive behavior to distract them from what feels like an uncontrollable internal experience. Uncomfortable with and most often afraid of their feelings, they tend to be emotionally reactive. Simply put, addicts use sex, food, gambling, alcohol, drugs, spending, and other stimulating or numbing combinations in an attempt to feel better and gain control over their feelings.

Addicts, frightened of the depth and intensity of feelings they have been suppressing for years will go to any length to avoid vulnerability. They engage in distorted thinking, which is termed *cognitive distortion*. Examples of distorted thinking are seeing things from an all-or-nothing perspective, difficulty perceiving options or choices, catastrophizing (seeing only the worst of outcomes), operating from "shoulds," and creating unrealistic expectations that only set themselves and others up for failure. The nature of distorted thinking creates further stress and painful feelings. To deal with this, addicts use the intense, familiar feelings provoked by sexual fantasy and sexual behavior to feel in control of deeper emotions, to feel power when they are feeling vulnerable, and to feel desirable when they are feeling needful. Many of their behaviors take advantage of somebody else's vulnerability or victimizing through intrusion or the use of power.

Escape, mood alteration, and validation are not the only reasons certain behaviors become addictive. Sometimes behaviors are used as a reward. Sex addicts do not usually have a healthy sense of how to reward themselves. Whether it comes from a core belief in their unworthiness or their entitlement, they have a belief system that others will not take care of them and they must do everything for themselves. That builds up resentments. Their resentments can be expressed in a sense of entitlement: *I deserve.* Whether it follows surviving stressful events, performing well, or doing a good job, sex addicts may believe they deserve to be rewarded, and sex is the manner in which they can do that for themselves.

[ADDICT]

I was so full of resentments and I took them into all of my relationships. I had been beat up a lot by my father and watched him beat my mom. Nothing I ever did was okay. By my mid-twenties I was into full-blown sex addiction with chronic masturbation, pornography, and escorts. As I'd get a new girlfriend, I'd try not to do those things. I always hinted that those things were a part of my past, never sharing the whole picture. I think I did that so that I could say I didn't lie when she eventually found out what I was doing. As much as it's possible for me to get outside of always thinking about just myself, I'd say I'm in love with my present girlfriend. But it's been only a few months and I'm already rationalizing that I deserve my fix. Those lifelong resentments only stay down so long, and I find that they sprout up like weeds in the cracks of a sidewalk. I use her like a balm, but no salve will take care of my anger. As painful as my life is, losing one loving woman after another because of my infidelities, it's too overwhelming for me to address my trauma history. So again I juggle hiding my secret life, and I can hear myself rationalizing how it is that I'm entitled and deserving of doing what I want when I want without having to think of anyone else.

Shared Traits

Many factors influence the way children develop. The most apparent is the socialization process that directs males more toward *acting-out* behaviors such as rage, substance abuse, and behavioral addictions (intensity and arousal behaviors), and females toward *acting-in* behaviors such as being nice, being tolerant, and not questioning others. When they feel overwhelmed, girls tend to respond by acting in through depression, anxiety, eating disorders, or sedating-type addictions, such as alcoholism or prescription pain pills. Men are much more apt to be culturally influenced to find a (false) sense of empowerment and esteem in their sexual prowess. Women are socialized to be timid and reserved in their sexual feelings and thoughts. Certainly this stereotyping is not always accurate; many women sexually act out in highly compulsive and self-defeating ways. And there are many men in coupleship with women sex addicts. But generally speaking, our culture has done much to influence who and how someone *acts out* or *acts in*. Many times people display both types of behavior. As you are considering whether any of your behaviors could also be addictive, know that addicts most often have significant underlying trauma and codependency issues.

Traits common to both the partner and addict include:

- Need for outside approval

- Fear of rejection and abandonment

- Inability to identify and ask for what you need

- Fear of conflict

- Feelings of inadequacy

- Inability to identify and express a wide range of feelings

- Shame-bound defenses, such as controlling, procrastination, victimhood, and so on

- Fear of specific feelings

- Adherence to rigidly ascribed roles learned in impaired family

[ADDICT]

I was so afraid of conflict. I was the peacekeeper type of guy. Peace at all costs—peace at work, peace with my wife—and I always felt inadequate, like I was never good enough. But I had my secrets. I would pay for women to do whatever I wanted. A lot of the time I had no expectations from them, I just wanted their attention.

I wasn't scared, and it was easier for me to perform sexually because they were strangers; they didn't need anything from me.

A household in which family members internalize their shame-based beliefs frequently trains a child to seek the approval of others, an approval he cannot give himself. Because of this the child becomes dependent on the positive response and praise of others to feel good about who he is. Both addicts and partners seek what is called *outer esteem*, which is esteem through others. They have not learned to internalize self-worth and value so they are in a perpetual state of looking for affirmation and validation. While women tend to seek outer esteem through their people pleasing, image management, and relationships, the sex addict comes to believe the only way to feel approval is through sexual activity. How much sex he scores, how many secrets he can get away with, how large his pornography collection is, how great he looks, and how much attention he can solicit—all are delusional ways to temporarily fill the emotional void.

The following story illustrates more fully the duality of codependency and addiction for a sex addict. It is also a reminder that much of what is identified to be codependent is in fact a trauma response. As said earlier in the book, codependency refers to the beliefs and behaviors learned in one's growing-up years, emotional and behavioral responses to traumatic stress.

[ADDICT]

By the time I was a teenager I was really angry, quietly angry. No matter what I did, the message I got from my father was that I wasn't good enough, and my mom was like a ghost: emotionally and mentally nonexistent. My father would rage at us kids and Mom would have this look on her face as if it was just something interesting. I would get violent spankings from my father. I was an impressionable kid who, like most kids, just wanted to be loved.

Today I am quite sure my father had affairs. People have told me they saw him with other women. And one person told me that when we were kids she saw an article about him being arrested for something of a sexual nature. My dad was abandoned young and had to go to work to support himself. He had a strong work ethic, and that was a positive trait I got from him. Mostly I feared him and our relationship was very poor due to his outbursts of temper, being unpredictable, and periodically drinking too much. My mom never knew what she wanted and would never directly make a statement. She was emotionally disconnected but she was my confidant, as I was hers.

We had our share of family secrets too. I didn't even know my paternal grandfather was alive until I was an adult and found out he had been locked away in a state mental institution for years due to wet brain, being a town drunk.

My primary belief of thinking that I was not good enough fueled my addictions, but I was also strongly influenced by a neighbor girl. When she was about twelve and I was nine or ten, she wanted to be sexual with me, but I was physically too young and couldn't. She was emotionally dominating, demanding, and intimidating, both sexually and physically. Looking back, I suspect she was being sexually abused because her knowledge of sex was too sophisticated for her age. Because of her, I didn't engage sexually with girls until I was older. I was always scared of them.

In college I was still scared of women and I let them be the pursuers. After a few sexual experiences, I found that the conquest gave me a sense of power and acceptance. But I had such a distorted perception about what women wanted or needed. My mother certainly didn't give me any positive direction, and my father only spoke of women in negative terms: "You marry the good girls and have sex with the bad girls."

From a young age this sex addict had a strong foundation for sexual addiction and codependency. Sex allowed him to ignore his pain; it provided a high and temporarily allowed him to feel important and valued. It was difficult for him to give it up because it had become his coping strategy. Sex kept him from drowning emotionally, and it was a quick fix. He experienced emotional abandonment from a very frightened boundary-less mother and an abusive father who acted out with alcohol and sex. Secrecy and addiction were multigenerational issues in his family. The way he describes his mother is the same way that he describes himself. He learned to not ask for what he wanted or needed and became conflict avoidant. He constantly sought outside approval with a strong need to look good. While treated for sex addiction, his early childhood experiences had to be addressed, as they could be significant relapse triggers.

Compartmentalizing

The highly developed defense of compartmentalizing, used by both addicts and their partners, is strongly influenced by childhood history. In our humanness we all compartmentalize, that is, we set aside feelings and thoughts about one moment while we are engaged in another. For example, if you have an argument with your teenage daughter prior to going to work, you may feel upset and think about it while you commute to your job. But when you walk through the door of your office, you mentally put it aside because you have work issues to attend to. We all do that and need to do it. But people who are raised with fear and shame practice the art of compartmentalizing more frequently, and its use is fueled from a place of greater need, often stemming from fear. It begins as a necessary defense but it becomes a skill that is practiced day in and day out, week in and week out, month after month, year after year. You can easily become masterful in the ability to live in two different worlds, or compartments, simultaneously.

Compartmentalizing starts at a young age. For example, you may listen to your parents argue night after night, but when you go to school the next day you act as if everything is fine; or you listen to your father molest your sister but you pretend it is not happening. Perhaps your mother told you how worthless you are, or you wonder why your father doesn't come home. How can you possibly talk to someone about these things? It's too painful. No one knows what your internal personal life is like or your thoughts or feelings. You learn the dysfunctional family rules: don't talk, don't feel, don't ask. While everyone compartmentalizes to some degree, it becomes a large part of emotional survivorship when you are raised in an environment of chronic loss, fear, and chaos. This ability to compartmentalize can set up many men to lead highly secretive, compartmentalized lives. It is a learned skill that enables this particular addiction.

[ADDICT]

I was very skilled at living in two worlds, or even three—home, work, and my outside world of sex. They were different compartments of my life that were never to meet. I was masterful at lying and simply couldn't allow myself to think about my work colleagues or wife finding out about my secret life. Since I was a kid I've been skilled at living in different worlds; I lived with terror at home, so I'd escape into my sexual fantasies, and then find relief at school. So it came easy. As I said, I was skilled.

[ADDICT]

Each day as I left my family home and went into the day, it was as if I crossed an invisible line. I didn't think twice about how what I was doing would affect my family life. I truly didn't think about it.

Such thinking on the part of the addict may be difficult to understand. His inability to empathize with your situation is a testament to the darkness and pervasiveness of addiction. It is also just as possible that as the addict has compartmentalized unsparingly, so have you.

[JACQUE]

As a young girl, I learned how to compartmentalize, keeping my sex abuse in a box, separate from the rest of my world. I'd tell myself this can't be happening to me, or this doesn't really matter, or it doesn't bother me. That's exactly what I would do around my husband's addiction. As a child, I found that school was a wonderful source of validation. As an adult, I've found that validation through work. Throwing myself into school and/or work helped me to stay separate from the pain and confusion in my life.

[THERESE]

I am so compartmentalized! Having kids helps—they keep me so busy. I dive into the Mom role. I think in some ways compartmentalizing has kept me from going crazy, but in the long run it allowed me to ignore what was happening in my marriage. Because I had no direction as to what to do about my situation, facing reality was too much. So like recipes clipped from a magazine, I filed the truth away as if I planned to get back to it later.

As a partner, you project to the world one image while internally living another, a well-developed habit you use to bury your head in the sand and pretend that everything is fine while the house burns down around you. While we all compartmentalize in the course of a day, this severe and chronic form of compartmentalizing supports you in the denial process.

* * *

Just as the addict in recovery needs to address the addictive nature of his behavior and learn how to get his needs met without being intrusive or exploitive of another person, both individuals in the coupleship need to examine how their belief systems, their emotional defenses, and their childhood wounding contribute to an unhealthy relationship. As you do that, your relationship has the opportunity to be one of choice rather than a relationship of script, repetition, or traumatic bonding. In this process you both learn how to develop empathy and compassion toward self and others. You learn how to develop healthy boundaries, greater emotional literacy, and the ability to handle your feelings without the need to engage in self-defeating behaviors.

Whether or not you have a lifelong commitment or are attracting the same man over and over, recognizing your pattern of how you choose a partner and contribute to the dance is critical to your ability to make healthy relationship decisions for yourself.

Reflective Thoughts and Questions

- Underline or highlight the parts of the stories with which you identify.

- In what ways did you experience abandonment in your childhood?

- To what degree have you engaged in trauma repetition? Explain.

- In what ways has abandonment influenced your behavior in your relationship(s)?

- What sexual messages did you hear growing up? Completing the following sentences may help.

    Sex means . . .

    I have the right to . . . (regarding sex)

    I don't have the right to . . . (regarding sex)

- What do you know about your partner's family history that may have contributed to his sexual acting out?

- What was important for you to learn in this chapter?

CHAPTER FOUR NOTES

1   Patrick Carnes, *The Betrayal Bond: Breaking Free of Exploitive Relationships* (Deerfield Beach, FL: Health Communications, Inc., 1997), 26.

2   Euripides (c. 485–406 BC)

3   Maureen Canning, *Lust, Anger, Love: Understanding Sexual Addiction and the Road to Healthy Intimacy* (Naperville, IL: Sourcebooks, 2008), 98.

CHAPTER FIVE

Learning the News

What should I do?

Do I want to know everything?

How can I show my face to those who may know?

How can I ever trust again?

Women learn about their partners' sexual acting out in a variety of ways. Perhaps you heard about your partner's behavior from a coworker, a friend, a neighbor, or a family member. It's possible someone told you inadvertently and didn't even realize what they said. Or perhaps the person knew full well what he or she was saying and did it out of respect for you. It could be that someone shared the information out of vindictiveness. You may have read about your partner's activities in the newspaper or saw him on television. Perhaps the police came to your door to take him away. His angry lover may have called and left a message or emailed you a letter and/or pictures. It is possible you happened upon your partner with his lover. You may have inadvertently found internet sex sites he bookmarked on the computer. Maybe he went to a treatment program for his addiction to gambling or drugs or alcohol and you suddenly found yourself sitting in a counselor's office, surprised to be learning about his sexual acting out. It's possible your child told you about something he or she saw. Sometimes women visit their doctor and learn they have a sexually transmitted disease. This news, whatever the setting or form of delivery, can be a bombshell. It can also be nothing more than a validation of what you've been suspecting.

[PARTNER]

The first time I learned he was acting out I had gone to his office after work with our baby in my arms just to see him. I had no idea I would find him in a compromised position with someone at work. I was numb. They laughed at me. I stayed with him several more years and had two more kids. He would never admit openly to what he was doing but I found the evidence: the hotel slips, the letters.

[PARTNER]

My husband had been in some intensive psychotherapy, and after one of his therapy retreats he came home an emotional mess and disclosed he was a sex addict. He told me it was a one-time ongoing affair with someone out of state. He told me it was over, and that was all that was said. Well, I had a history of sex abuse as a child and to use the word "sex addict" was so scary. Sex addict, sex abuser, sexual molester—were they all one and the same? I didn't know what to think, so I focused on what he said about this affair being over and I thought, *Good, it's over with,* and locked it up in some mental container in my head to not think about it. But what I did not know for a long time was he was acting out more and more.

[PARTNER]

Because I was suspicious, I went searching for proof and found his journal, which was the darkest day of my life. I read about affairs that had been going on for years, for one hour, one night, several months, and multiple affairs at the same time. I thought I would die. I actually thought about suicide. I was overwhelmed and wanted a divorce. He went to treatment. I didn't hear any additional information. I really got it all in his journal so there was nothing more to add. As hard as it is to know—and I did need to know, to get to where we are today—that was not the way to find out. I wish it had been a structured therapeutic disclosure.

Every discovery is a trauma-inducing event. Often partners become overwhelmed and go into a freeze state putting their heads into the sand for years. Others have suicidal thoughts and often think of dying. Needless to say it's a horrific time, a time of great darkness.

When you first hear the news, you may only take in a piece of the whole picture. It's likely that even if you are aware of the severity of the acting out, you may not view it as an addiction from which one recovers, but more like something that men just do. You may believe if the man feels guilty enough, he will just stop. Your response may be one of shame, guilt, fear, and rage, and very often you have no safe environment to express these feelings or even begin to understand the ramifications of what is occurring. Even with the very real threat of leaving the relationship or getting a divorce, unless the addict is in a treatment/recovery program for sex addiction, you are probably not hearing the full extent of his behavior. Therefore, neither you nor he is seeing its addictive nature. While some women are genuinely unaware of the behavior at the time they hear the news, most suspect or are somewhat aware of the acting out. And many, when they do find out, say they would prefer not knowing. In the long run, it is my professional bias that you will benefit more from knowing about his behavior than not. Addictive behavior flourishes in isolation and secrecy. It is a therapeutic tenet that secrets not only interfere with recovery, they preclude the possibility of recovery and they will fuel relapse. As difficult as it is for him to disclose the extent of his behavior and for you to hear it, it is a vital aspect of the recovery process both for you individually and for your relationship.

The value of knowing the truth is that it reinforces trust in your own perceptions and allows you to deal honestly with the relationship. Knowing the truth gives the relationship the potential for an honest foundation. You deserve to have the information to make objective choices about whether or not you want to continue in the relationship and/or go through the journey of potential recovery with him.

Disclosure

At the time of initial awareness, in the heat of rage or the pain of shame, you may demand to know everything. Whether you are at home, in a car, in a motel room, or in a public place, it doesn't matter to you—you want to know and you want to know now.

[PARTNER]

My boyfriend disclosed all right—I discovered him all over the internet. That was my experience with disclosure.

[PARTNER]

Well, I thought my husband disclosed, meaning he told me about the pornography. But later he told me about the chat rooms and then he told me about the woman at work. I have been disclosed to a lot.

[PARTNER]

My husband did this disclosure and we didn't have any facilitation. I was so angry I think I scared him, and because I insisted, he told me lots of details. I kept screaming that if he wanted me to stay he had to tell me everything, so unfortunately I got everything, including her clothes size and color of hair and eyes. I wanted to know exactly which internet sites he was on. I wanted to know what they did when they had dates, where they had gone, etc. So what did I do with that? I made him take me to the places he took her. For whatever reason, he mostly acted out with redheads, and so being a brunette I quickly colored my hair red. I had him buy me the exact presents he bought the other women. Well, none of this did anything for me or him. It just kept me wound up and him crazy.

These women certainly "got the news," in a variety of ways but that's not what I'm talking about here. The word *disclosure* is a therapeutic term that describes a structured conversation mediated by a professional counselor who provides both physical and emotional safety, wherein the addict shares (discloses) the extent of his sexual acting-out behavior. While it is emotionally difficult, when it's done in a manner that offers support to both of you, it has the potential to lessen the craziness you have been experiencing and provide much-needed validation to your suspicions.

In a professionally mediated disclosure process the standard practice is for the generalities—not the specifics—of the acting-out behavior be disclosed. Some partners insist on all the details down to the color of a lover's clothing. The Women of the Lodge refer to that as *pain shopping.* You seek the details, but being privy to minute details only tends to help you stay obsessed and reactive, resulting in more pain and anxiety.

Essentially you are taking the detailed information and recycling it. Traumatized by knowing his every behavior, you re-traumatize yourself. Some women don't want to know anything about what happened. They just want to hear that the behavior has stopped. To assume the behavior has stopped because it has been exposed is denial. Seeing only one piece of the picture maintains your denial about the seriousness and extent of the problem. Ignorance is not bliss.

When you know the bigger picture it may seem like your relationship is in even more trouble than you previously thought. Yet, addiction thrives in secrecy. Truth is the only way intimacy is ever truly achieved. There is no doubt that this is a time of intense feelings and great uncertainty, but disclosure levels the playing field. Since you are no longer in the dark, you are in a better position to know how to go forward and make informed decisions. I strongly recommend that you and your partner work through the disclosure with therapists trained and certified in working with couples impacted by sex addiction. (See Helpful Resources in the back of this book.)

[THERESE]

I agreed to the disclosure, after all it seemed that we were both working up to it with our separate therapists. I really wanted to hear what he had to say, yet, I still wasn't sure. I knew the pretending had to stop. Just being ready to try to move on wherever we went in our relationship made it easier for me to hear. Oh, I hated him in the moment. I couldn't look at him, though I hung on to every word. I did ask a couple of questions. It was important for me to know if any of our family knew of this and to know the last time he was on the internet. I heard him talk about what he was going to do to stop this behavior, but what impacted me was how much more serious this was than I had guessed.

[PARTNER]

I'd already knew a lot about my partner's behavior before we had this formal disclosure, but it was helpful for me to hear it in a more level way. It wasn't so emotional now. I knew we were having this conversation because we were trying to keep our marriage and I am hopeful that we will, but I'm aware he and I both have a lot of work to do.

For a disclosure to be helpful and to lessen furthering greater trauma, there are suggested prerequisites.

1. Addict is demonstrating commitment to stop all acting-out behavior (this means actively involved in some form of treatment/recovery practice).
2. Addict needs foundation in recovery. Therapist assesses the addict's ability to be honest, his emotional strength, his understanding of his behavior and makes recommendation for timing.
3. Partner needs understanding of sex addiction, that the behavior not about the partner, and garnering understanding of traumatic responses.
4. Boundaries for discussion agreed upon. There are established boundaries as to the content, and to self-care. Listening and speaking boundaries are explained, so neither party is subject to being victimized. Both containment and protection boundaries will be in place. Both parties able to demonstrate emotional regulation.

5. Partner has established support. Support system informed when the disclosure will take place. Because it is difficult to remain objective, family and friends often not the best support. Your best support may be a peer group of others in recovery

6. Support is available to both individuals before, during, and after disclosures

Suggested generalities to be shared in disclosure are:

1. In what type(s) of behavior was he engaged? (For example, extramarital affairs, prostitution, pornography, voyeurism, masturbation, fetishes, and so on.)
2. How long has he been acting out?
3. Is there a possibility that either of you is at risk of sexually transmitted diseases? Will his acting-out behavior affect your health?
4. Have the family finances been impacted? How has the money been acquired, and how much has been spent to engage in the behavior?
5. Are there any legal issues, such as the possibility of other children or legally binding arrangements with others? (Owning property with a mistress, outstanding warrants, pending court action, and so on.)
6. Did he engage in any behaviors with friends, family members, or other individuals known to you?

Most sex addiction experts believe disclosure is beneficial to the addict, the partner, and the coupleship. Truth telling is an important component in restoring trust.

For the partner, this type of disclosure has the potential to:

• Allow for an adult-to-adult relationship on an equal basis

• Empower her with the truth

- Give her the ability to make informed choices based on the truth

- Allow her to embrace recovery

For the addict, it:

- Reinforces accountability in his recovery

- Reinforces honesty with others and self

- Facilitates the letting go of his shame

For both, it begins the opportunity to:

- Break the addictive system

- Heal the relationship

[ADDICT]

I was pushed into telling my partner by my counselor. I went to treatment only because I knew this time she would really leave me. I didn't really get what it meant to be an addict. When questioned in treatment, I was honest about what I had been doing. But I didn't want to tell her because I knew she would be mad and I would disappoint her. I knew deep down she was the best person ever in my life. I knew she loved me when I couldn't and hadn't been able to love myself. I didn't want her to see the terrible person I was. But I put my trust in those counselors, and today I believe it was important to put the information into the light—it is what allowed us to move forward.

[ADDICT]

I'm sitting in front of the woman I married and she can't look at me. She seems so fragile, and I tell her all of these things about myself. I felt worse than an animal that lives underground. I felt I didn't deserve her. I so didn't want her to leave me but knew she might. I had to do this for us to have a chance.

The impact of planned and mediated disclosures vary, but again, if working with skilled sex addiction and partner trained therapists, partners will find a mediated disclosure was needed to go forward with healing.

THE DRIBBLING EFFECT

Even when you participate in a mediated disclosure, and you think you've been told the whole story, many partners experience what I call the "dribbling effect." You think you have been told everything, and then with time more and more information gradually reveals itself.

[PARTNER]

As we sat in a therapist's office and he told me what had been going on throughout our entire marriage, I kept asking him if that was all, had he told me everything. He swore that was it. He was crying, asking me not to leave. I told myself somehow I would cope with this.

Somehow we could find a way to go forward now that I knew. But then over the next two years I would find out more. He was no longer acting out but he hadn't told me a lot of the real story at the supposed time of disclosure. I would find out more because I found pictures when I was in his office. I found out more when I was reviewing some retirement accounts. I found out more when he told me one day he had something else he needed to tell me. It was about his once being involved with a woman I knew who was moving back to our community. Each time I got more information, it was a setback for me. I honestly believe that as painful as it would have been, it would have been better for me to know everything all at once. He would tell me he had told me all, and then more kept coming. It made it hard to believe there wasn't yet more to come.

Even when working with a counselor and encouraged to be as honest as possible, he may not be prepared to be totally honest. Sometimes his shame is so great he is only emotionally equipped to share some information; other times he may consciously or unconsciously be protecting his stash; or he may think disclosing additional information will be the deal breaker for the coupleship and he is too scared to take that chance.

It's also possible that at the time of disclosure an addict may not fully remember some of his past behaviors. Addicts are very skilled in compartmentalizing their behaviors and have learned to detach from them often within hours, if not minutes, after engaging. So when months and often years pass, some behaviors may be quite distant from his consciousness. To live with the shame, he has learned how to push aside specific memories and details.

As those memories are triggered (by a conversation, by being in a specific place, or while watching a movie, for example), he is then confronted with how he is going to reveal this information to you. Either he shares it and risks you believing he has deliberately been deceiving you, or he says nothing and you inadvertently discover the information.

No doubt, this dribbling disclosure is debilitating to building trust. But if you and he are engaged in recovery practices, you can get through this excruciating phase. I strongly suggest that you take any new information that has dribbled out after a planned and mediated disclosure to a counselor to facilitate healthy discussion and accountability.

After Disclosure

Hearing the news is painful and your response may vary from relief that finally your perceptions and your senses are validated to humiliation, shame, rage, disbelief, and back again. This emotional roller coaster can last for days and even weeks. You may be asking, "What now? Just because he's finally honest doesn't make everything okay." It's not okay—it hurts, and it hurts deeply.

Depending on the extent of the behavior and your level of surprise the first few days and weeks after disclosure can be very overwhelming. Some women are not so overwhelmed as much as they are relieved to hear the truth, or have their suspicions validated. After taking in the information, remember that you do have choices, and it is important that you ascertain what you need as far as contact and distance are concerned. For the moment, make no major decisions other than those that involve your safety. Most partners need time apart from the addict. It may be an hour, a few hours, one night, a few days, or even longer. You may choose to sleep separately for a while or not even stay in the same house. While the addict may perceive this as punishing behavior, healthy boundaries are about honoring the pain you feel and what you need at this time for your own emotional safety.

You may feel confused about boundaries and ultimatums. You aren't setting boundaries to punish him, you set them to honor and protect yourself, to help you feel safe and confident so that you can heal.

Whether the disclosure came as a surprise or was professionally mediated—or perhaps it was both—there are likely more additional issues to be attended to as a consequence of hearing the news. There are often immediate problems that range from financial, to legal, to public exposure issues, etc. You also have other areas of your life that need your time, such as work or school, raising children or even grandchildren, and other activities. It's best to take things one step at a time. Take a deep breath, ask for guidance, and do the next indicated step. Then breathe again, ask for guidance, and move forward again—one step at a time.

GETTING TESTED FOR STDS

Regardless of how you learn the news, it is vital to your health that you get tested for all sexually transmitted diseases. Even if you believe your partner had no physical contact with another person—because he was engaged in voyeurism, exhibitionism, or cyber sex—this step is essential. It's a healthy precaution, as you may not yet know the full extent of the acting out, and it may be more than he is telling you. This is another dark moment in the process of living with sexual compulsivity. Most partners say that being tested is humiliating, and for many it evokes incredible anger and despair. Nevertheless, your responsibility to yourself is a priority. This is a positive step in your self-care and your healing.

[PARTNER]

Here I am looking at this questionnaire in the doctor's office. Do I use IV drugs? Do I have multiple sex partners? Do I practice unsafe sex? Do I engage in unusual sex? Then I see the "Other" box in which I get to write, "My husband of twelve years has sex with prostitutes and then comes home to me." I want to scream. I want to die. I want to tear his eyes out. And instead I hold my head up and act like this is an everyday occurrence. Funny, maybe it has been.

[PARTNER]

I'm sitting in my doctor's office and she asks me if I'm okay, as obviously I don't look okay. My face is bloated and my eyes are red from crying and I tell her I need to be tested for STDs because my husband is a sex addict and I'm really not sure I know who he has been with. I then burst into sobs and she simply takes my hands in hers and waits until I'm done crying. Then, without any judgment but with great compassion, she tells me we will find out what we need to know.

Shame and/or denial can prevent or stall you from being tested. You might be thinking, *My partner would not engage in something that would cause me to develop a chronic or even fatal health problem. And if he did, of course he would tell me.* But being tested is necessary and will relieve or confirm any thoughts about possible exposure.

[PARTNER]

My first exposure to a STD was pretty significant, as it threatened the welfare of our unborn child. I was having herpes outbreaks during my pregnancy and we had a serious talk about a caesarean section to deliver the baby safely. I had never had herpes until after I had been with my husband for a few years. I told myself it couldn't be from him, but I also knew I had not been exposed to anyone else.

[PARTNER]

When I became aware of the extent of his acting out, I don't know if I felt more anger about anything other than the fact that he would thoughtlessly risk my health and even my life with unsafe sex. How could he do that to anyone, especially me, his wife? Today I get that he just didn't think about that and that it is a part of the addiction. In spite of being terrified, I did not get tested because I had a life insurance physical exam coming up and knew there would be some blood work that would verify if I had HIV or another sexually transmitted disease. Even after the exam, as scared as I was awaiting the results, I was so ashamed I couldn't talk to anyone about it.

[PARTNER]

I discovered during my husband's disclosure that his way of reassuring himself that he was safe was by donating blood, because part of the blood donation screening process is testing for HIV. How could he be so careless with his and my safety? To stoop to those bizarre levels of justification and denial around what he was doing to us was incomprehensible to me.

Again, being tested is an act of self-care. You don't have to explain your circumstances to anybody, not the nurse, not the doctor. Just tell the physician you have a need to be checked for all sexually transmitted diseases.

BEING SEXUAL AFTER DISCLOSURE
How can you be sexual with your partner who has betrayed you?

If you are *not* sexual with him, are you giving him justification to act out again? If you *are* sexual with him, are you crazy to even want to be with him? These are normal and expected questions at this stage. There is a lot of emotional intensity attached to these concerns.

First, you are not giving him justification to act out if you do not want to be sexual right now. If he is serious about wanting a healthy relationship with you, he will honor this boundary. Remember, addicts use whatever they can to justify their behavior. It is not your responsibility to control him. If you find yourself wanting to be sexual after hearing the disclosure and that surprises you, know that for some people this desire to be sexual is a form of validation that they are still desirable. For him, sex is the answer to most things, and his desire for sex with you may be to garner assurance that you still love him and won't leave him. The consuming desire to be sexual by either of you in the face of crisis, often referred to as the *honeymoon effect,* is an attempt to reaffirm that all will be okay. Unfortunately, it only offers a temporary and false sense of security, an illusion of safety. This doesn't mean that the relationship isn't going to work. It is a combination of time with active recovery practices that has the potential to sustain the relationship.

Answering the following questions as honestly as you can will help you recognize your motives and help you decide whether or not you are ready to be sexual with your partner.

- Do I want to be sexual out of fear he will go elsewhere if I am not?

- Do I think I will be able to control his behavior if I am sexual with him?

- Do I believe having sex reaffirms he still loves me?

- Do I withhold sex as a way of punishing him?

- Do I not want to be sexual with him because I don't feel the intimacy sex would imply?

To aid in this initial decision, know that nearly all sex addiction specialists recommend an initial ninety-day period of no sexual behavior in early recovery. The purpose of this abstinence contract, which is really a verbal agreement, is not to punish either the addict or you, but to help the addict learn how to better articulate his feelings and thoughts without using sex as a medicator or fix. It is essential for him to learn new skills for getting his emotional and relational needs met. This ninety-day sabbatical also affords you time to begin your healing. While some women say the sex between them and their partner is still good, this is not a time-out that focuses on the physicality of sex but a break from the physical act to rebuild trust, emotional intimacy, and safety in your relationship. Also know there is nothing particularly magical at ninety days. The pain may still be so great, and recovery behavior so new that you need more time before you are ready to pursue sexual intimacy. The coupleship needs emotional intimacy before sexual intimacy feels safe. There are many issues that will influence one's readiness, and it is very likely the idea of healthy sexuality is so foreign it needs to be navigated with a therapist.

When being sexual with your partner is an option for you it is critical that you approach it from a place of strength.

Should I Stay or Should I Leave?

Many women have threatened to leave a relationship if their suspicions are validated or the behavior reoccurs; some do leave, while others, in spite of their threats, do not. If family and friends know of your situation, they may encourage you either to leave or to disregard his behavior and stay. Regardless of past threats, to leave or stay is a decision that you want to make from a position of inner strength, not because of emotional reactivity (a time of emotional overload interfering with the ability to think through the situation clearly). If you are just beginning your own recovery, you don't have to make such a major decision right now. When you feel as if your head and heart are spinning, make as few life-changing decisions as you can. It is easy to believe that the problem is totally him and that leaving him or getting a divorce is the quick, simple solution: *If he was just out of my life, it would be such a relief.* But quitting the relationship out of spite causes more problems in the long run. I'm not saying you should stay in the relationship. I'm saying if you take some time, things will become clearer. When you immerse yourself in finding your voice and your strengths and can objectively assess how seriously your partner is engaging in his recovery practices, you will have clarity.

[PARTNER]

With the last discovery, and they have been going on for over thirty-eight years, I knew I was leaving. And he knew it too. I always threatened but this was different. I was really done. But he did what he could. He did what he never did before. He sought help and he sought the right help. I was honest, I told him I just couldn't stay but I needed time. I think he thought because I didn't move out right away he had a chance. I even attended therapy sessions with him. I wanted help to understand, and I wanted him to feel I supported his recovery. But I didn't feel an ounce of love anymore. I didn't want to spend the rest of my life with him even if he was totally changed. It took me about a year and half, but I did leave. He is the father of my children and I hope he embraces recovery. For me, I have a lot to heal from.

[PARTNER]

It's odd because I knew of some of my husband's behavior and suspected even more. But it wasn't until a counselor guided us in a disclosure process that I insisted upon some level of separation. I asked that at least for a few nights he stay with a friend or at least outside of the house. I couldn't make a decision past just a few days. After those few days, it felt okay for him to come back home. We have two young children and we both thought that they needed to see him. So for the next few weeks, I simply asked that he sleep in a different room.

We managed to have dinner together with the kids. Our conversation at home was very superficial. Our much-needed serious conversations were with a counselor. I was also quickly directed to a women's group where I did a lot of talking that I needed to do. But I also heard a lot of things that I needed to hear. While I was still incredibly hurt, angry, and unsure, we gradually resumed sleeping in the same bed. What I came to realize is that I didn't want to "throw the baby out with the bath water." I believe there is hope.

When women leave with spite, they take their confusion, righteous anger, blame, and pain with them, contaminating all aspects of their lives. It impacts how they feel about themselves, how they relate to others, and their parenting skills. It increases the likelihood of not completing the grief process or addressing any family of origin dynamics. As much as you vow and can't believe you'd ever repeat this experience, not addressing these issues sets you up for trauma repetition.

[PARTNER]

After three years of my husband having countless affairs and berating me sexually, I left him for another man. What I didn't know was that this new guy already had a girlfriend at the time.

So sure enough, it was happening again. But I was determined to make this relationship work, thinking that somehow I was just a failure at relationships. After a couple of years, he left me. I took a break from relationships for a while. Feeling better about myself, I then met another man and after a year of dating we married. Within days of my wedding I was a raving lunatic, totally searching for "the other woman." I nearly drove my new husband away. He was the one who told me I should go address my issues. He called them mine—not my previous husband's problems. I was clearly taking my fears of abandonment, my anger, and my pain from my previous relationship and dumping them into my new relationship.

MAKING THE DECISION

In the long run, the decision to stay or leave often involves incremental steps to garner a stronger foundation to make that decision.

[SARA]

Over the years, in spite of my suspicions and even some knowledge, I stayed in the marriage because I craved safety more than anything. But when we had a real name for it, when he and I both recognized it was sex addiction, by then there was so much muddy water under the bridge that the additional knowledge was too much. I needed a time-out. I pretty much knew that right away. I couldn't contain my anger in his presence, and I had so much to deal with—my breast cancer in particular. A separation was suddenly a very clear and viable option. But he was motivated and getting the kind of help he had needed for years. I didn't know for sure what I wanted. The time-out gave me clarity and I could go forward. After nearly a year of separation, we both arrived at the same decision: since we had been together in the addiction, we wanted to try being together in recovery.

Sara realizes that she and her husband didn't have the opportunity to know what was possible in their relationship in a healthy way because for years he was trapped in his addiction and she in her trauma. The timing of learning about the depth of betrayal was complicated as she was also battling cancer. She knew herself well enough to know that her judgment about any decisions she would need to make regarding her physical care and her marriage was severely impaired by the depth of her anger. The anger was so great that she wanted the physical separation; she wanted time with herself so she wasn't in a state of reactivity. She needed to gain clarity.

After months of separation she was now experiencing her husband differently. Even more important to her, she was experiencing herself differently and she wanted to see if there was potential for them as a couple. She understood that there were no assurances about her husband's behavior, but she saw a commitment on his part to be in therapy and attend workshops and twelve-step meetings for his sex addiction. She also experienced him differently in his communication. She didn't see or feel any of the old behavior. This gave her hope. But, more important, she was learning a lot about herself in her own therapy process. She realized she had a self-destructive pattern with men and that it was not about her choosing a different man but about being different herself. She was finding her voice in her ability to know what she wanted and needed; she was learning to own that verbally. She was learning about boundaries. She was learning to focus on herself more and to act from a place of self-care instead of self-protection.

THERAPEUTIC SEPARATION

The process Sara has described is a *therapeutic separation*. It is not unusual to want some degree of separation to sort out your thoughts and feelings. Best facilitated by a therapist or counselor, together you and your partner agree to a separation for a specific amount of time. Then you will come back together to renegotiate the terms of the relationship at the end of that time. Significant to this process is that each of you has a specific plan about what you will be addressing during this separation period. For example, you commit to work with a therapist on childhood issues once a week, you agree to read specific books related to partner betrayal, he agrees to go to a treatment program, or he agrees to end certain relationships. You will also make decisions as to what type and amount of contact you will have during this time and what specific financial and parenting responsibilities are maintained.

The following couple decided to take a therapeutic separation very soon after the initial disclosure. Being together was simply not an option for them.

[PARTNER]

By the time my husband went to treatment for his sex addiction, I wanted a divorce. Nonetheless I agreed to participate in the therapy process they had for family members. Our relationship was so antagonistic and acrimonious that we both agreed to an immediate separation. I really thought we would divorce. But I followed the therapist's advice and made no legal decisions. I used this time to focus on myself and try to figure out what I wanted and more of who I was. I had so much anger long before this marriage. Overall,

I liked our separation; I found a freedom. It felt better than being together. While we thought it would be a three-month separation, it was actually a year. We both attended twelve-step programs, and both of us did a lot of therapy. It took a lot of discussion for me to have ownership of myself and some independence of him. After a year we got back together, but I still wasn't convinced it would work. Well, here we are twelve years later. I never would have imagined we would be the people we are today. We committed ourselves individually to our respective therapy processes and by doing so came together as a family.

The next example of therapeutic separation is less acrimonious. This couple believes therapeutic separation allowed them to learn more of what they needed individually, separate from each other, to allow them a healthier relationship down the road.

[PARTNER]

My husband and I have been in recovery for many years, he regarding pornography and myself for betrayal trauma and codependency. During this time he has had a few relapses. In our seventh year of recovery his acting out escalated.

He was going to massage parlors and having physical contact. I requested that he sleep in a separate bedroom for a few nights. I was angry, scared, and confused, and I didn't feel I could honor him or myself by sharing the same bed. Due to his relapse behavior, our counselor recommended shifting the dynamics in our coupleship with a ninety-day therapeutic separation. The first thirty days, outside of counseling, we would have no contact unless there was a physical emergency. The next thirty days would be renegotiated. Immediately, I felt scared as to what this meant for our marriage. We had been married for twenty-six years; he is my best friend. Yet I understood that something had to change. I didn't want to keep living a life of his acting out. I cried a lot during the first few weeks. The accumulation of fear, sadness, and not knowing where our marriage was headed worried me. But clearly both of us found the separation helpful. He is confronting some major underlying issues that with my presence were being glossed over, particularly owning his anger. I also see how enmeshed we were, to the point of being unhealthy. In just a short period of time I see how, as individuals and as a couple, we will be healthier and have a greater possibility of recovery.

[JACQUE]

We had a therapeutic separation a couple years after we began recovery. He had a slip in his sexual sobriety and it was my sponsor who suggested to me that a time-out may be what I need to do for me. The separation coincided with his decision to seek treatment for his loss and trauma issues, which were triggering relapse. One of the things I worked on most for myself during this time was what life would be like if I chose to divorce.

While I did not make the decision to divorce, it was an important issue to explore. It was very empowering. I realized that even with a divorce I could go on and live my life. I would feel great loss but the idea of being by myself was no longer so frightening. I had spent my whole life wanting to be safe and had given my sense of safety over to men who violated or betrayed me. I finally was really getting the idea that I had the ability and the responsibility to make myself safe. Well, now a few years have passed. We have chosen to stay together and I am hopeful for our relationship. Today my choice to stay is from a place of strength, not fear.

[JENNY]

After one and a half years of attempting recovery practices, my husband and I pursued a therapeutic separation that ultimately preceded our divorce. To say the least, we were having a rocky time. I was working so hard to figure out who I was and what I needed. I think that was confusing to him. I think he thought that if he just said he wasn't acting out anymore, everything would be okay. But the relationship had not been okay on most levels for years. So I just kept moving forward in terms of knowing that I needed a life other than being reactive to him. As I stayed fervent in my recovery process, he eventually stopped all of his counseling. Most of our core issues were still unresolved. I had learned so much about healthy relationships that I knew that I could not be in a relationship that didn't practice recovery. I was committed to becoming healed, not only for my benefit, but for the long-term benefit of my kids as well. My spiritual healing was very strong and with trusted friends for support, I knew what I needed to do. I never thought I would ever be divorced or be the one to file for one. In my marriage my

> husband was always the one threatening to divorce
> me! While I was scared, I made the decision from
> a position of strength.

Although Jenny chose to divorce her husband after a therapeutic separation, many couples reenter their renegotiated marriages successfully. For many couples, structured time out with terms and goals often secures their coupleship.

It is important that you do what works for you. Do what you think is healthiest for you. Your best determination will come from a place of strength, not from fear or shame or rage.

Am I Crazy to Love Him?

In your healing journey it is normal to experience a multitude of feelings and, often, contradictory ones. You may hate him one moment, love him the next, be enraged another, and then feel profound sadness. But no, you aren't crazy for still feeling love. You may honor valued history together and treasure what you experience to be honest times. Others may certainly tell you you're crazy. Then some partners are so angry, tired, and despairing they can't fathom the thought of still loving the addict. But don't confuse your loving feelings with not being free to be angry or not having a voice. These feelings are yours—yours to own without having to justify or explain. Remember, though, that while love is often unconditional, healthy relationships are not. To make your relationship work you need to establish conditions. It will take time to sort out the basis of your love, its strength and foundation.

Learning the news, whether it's done in a formal disclosure process, a media story, or an inadvertent mishap, can make you feel like your heart has been ripped out of your chest. The intensity and waves of emotion seem relentless and never-ending. Yet when you allow yourself the opportunity to be witnessed, validated, and led by others who have been there and found a path out of this dark time, you will find the strength to take the self-care actions that are a part of your healing. There are a lot of questions at this stage. Your head may feel as if it is exploding or you may be absolutely numb—probably both—but you will find answers. It is my hope that you are already finding direction and will continue to do so as you read on.

Reflective Thoughts and Questions

- How did you initially become aware or suspicious of your partner's behavior?

- What are your thoughts and feelings about further disclosure with a therapist?

- Have you experienced the dribbling effect? If so, what has that been like for you?

- Have you been, and/or are you willing to be, tested for sexually transmitted diseases?

- Would a short-term celibacy contract be helpful to you? If so, explain. Do you see the value of it for your partner?

- What was important for you to learn in this chapter?

CHAPTER SIX

What Do You Tell Your Children?

My kids are asking:

Did I do something wrong?

Do you still love each other?

What's wrong with Dad?

Talking with your children about sexually addictive behavior is undoubtedly a situation that no parent wants to face. Parents seldom want to share their secrets, their pain, or their betrayal with their children. You don't want your children to suffer; you want to protect them from pain. Yet all members of a family are affected by the trauma of sexual betrayal. Healthy communication and recovery practices make it possible to clear up any confusion your children experience and to create a greater sense of emotional safety.

It isn't just about family; your children already live in a highly sexualized culture. They are ruthlessly bombarded with sexual messages through the media, television, music, and the internet. Sex represents power and desirability. Consequently, "good enough" parenting involves not only healthy modeling of sexual expression but discussing sexual issues with children earlier than in generations past. But when sexual addiction operates within a family, the need for dialogue about sexuality emerges even sooner and more urgently than parents would usually choose. Kids often sense things aren't right at home. Disclosure to children helps them to understand why.

Children's Reactions

Many years ago, Stefanie Carnes, PhD and Diane Dillon, MA, and I developed a questionnaire that we administered to eighty-nine children who had a sexually addicted parent. (Twenty-two of these children were under the age of eighteen; the others were of adult age.) We wanted to learn from these children what they knew about their parent's sexual acting out and how they were told about it. We discovered that many of the children already knew about the acting out or had suspicions about it before their parents disclosed to them.[1] Since that time, what we learned has been repeatedly validated in clinical work.

As much as parents wish to protect children from their own mistakes or hurtful behaviors, keeping secrets does not provide the sought-after protection. Sixty of eighty-nine respondents indicated they knew about their parent's behavior prior to disclosure. Here is a sampling of some of the responses we received:

> "I was surprised that my mother was not aware that I knew. I carried this secret with me my entire adolescence!"

> "I knew. I had read my father's diary. It was quite a shock. I told my best friend but I never told anyone else."

> "Sure, I would rather have not known about any of this. I don't think any of us who have had this

experience want to know this stuff. But that is impossible because in my case I was living in a house with two addicts: my father who was a sex addict, and my mother who was addicted to him."

"I don't know which part is the most unfair, that he is doing what he does or that he doesn't know I am like the fairy princess who has to keep the knight's honor clean."

"I knew my dad had this woman friend; he would have me with him in the car sometimes when he called her. And I just knew he shouldn't be talking to her the way he did."

Of twenty-nine respondents who were asked directly if they were glad they were told about their parent's behavior, twenty responded affirmatively. Yet they also said they did not like the actual moment of learning it was true. When questioned further, they said they did not want their beliefs or suspicions to be true. At the time of the disclosure, many experienced anger: anger for the pain to the other parent, anger for the embarrassment, but predominantly anger over their lives having been turned upside down. They were often fearful of the financial ramifications.

"I felt like I wanted to punch them. But I just sat there."

"My dad was going on about his being a sex addict and treatment and steps and other stuff that I couldn't care less about, and the word 'bankruptcy' came up because at the time we were being sued, and that really struck a chord with me. What did that mean for me? Would I lose my chance to go to college?"

For many of the children we evaluated, the term sex addiction created a picture of their parent being a pervert or a child molester.

They frequently found themselves in fear of a parent whom they had previously trusted.

> "I felt sick, horrified. What are other people going to think? Can I be left home alone with him?"

Confusion was a predominant feeling the children experienced with the disclosure.

> "I was only seven! I was too little to understand. And now we had to move and I had to leave my friends. That is what I understood. The last thing I needed was to feel different from other kids."

> "I was really too young (eleven). I didn't know much about sex and it was foreign. I really couldn't imagine my dad doing the things he did and that was hard for me."

> "This made my relationship with my dad very awkward when I didn't find it that way before. I felt very uncomfortable being left alone with him."

The children often became compliant or reached out to emotionally take care of their parent(s). Even when they knew what their parent did was not okay, they felt a need to be protective of one or both of their parents.

> "I knew my dad was being forced to tell me. If he didn't tell me, my stepmother would have. She was really angry and was divorcing him. He was crying and so embarrassed. I didn't know what to do or feel—mostly I felt sorry for him. He really was my only safe parent, and I knew what he did was supposed to be bad, but how could I be angry? I was more scared I would lose him."

> "I felt like I had to defend and protect my dad."

> "My mom was crying so hard, I just wanted her
> to stop. I wanted to do anything to make her feel
> better."

It is not uncommon for children to take sides. They may blame one or both parents.

> "Maybe if my mom wasn't always so angry with
> my dad he wouldn't have done what he did."

> "My dad is really a good guy so I don't know why
> Mom is making such a big deal of this."

> "No one should have boyfriends or girlfriends
> when they are married. That just isn't the way it
> is supposed to be. My dad really hurt my mom and
> that's not right!"

Some of the children said they had no awareness of the behavior until disclosure was made to them, and then they were shocked. They said that to hear about the behavior was a negative experience. We don't know if their negative experience was due to the behavior's impact on their lives because the parents were now visibly reacting to the consequences, or the children's confusion as to what it meant about their parent and how they understood the words *sex addiction*. While most parents would like to believe their children are unaware, in fact, many children said they either sensed or knew.

While some children were shocked and confused by the disclosure, some found immediate relief and/or validation. They finally understood why they were feeling confused, fearful, or anxious.

> "I was initially so shocked, my stomach kind of
> dropped. I was thinking, *I can't believe I am hearing this.*
> It just blew me away and at the same time incredible
> relief, wow!"

"I was not crazy. I had known all along!"

"I think a lot of parents think that their kids don't know. I think that is a huge mistake. We know almost everything our parents do. We aren't stupid. We may not know exactly what it is but we know enough to wonder, *Why is Mom or Dad doing this?* I think disclosure is a good thing."

Rationale for Disclosure to Children

So the question is: why would you even tell your children? There is no discounting the difficulty of your decision to disclose. I know there is a lot to consider: their ages, the setting, the timing, who tells them, and how much to tell. Let me offer four pertinent reasons to disclose to children.

1. **Validation**

   Disclosure validates what the children know. Having their unspoken perceptions validated takes away the craziness of knowing but at the same time not knowing. It diminishes the additional shame and anxiety that comes with secrecy.

2. **Exposure**

   Children may find out anyway. Often other family members, particularly a sibling, or other children in the neighborhood or at school know and may deliberately or inadvertently tell them. Thoughtful disclosure can be offered in a healthy manner to counteract a mean-spirited or otherwise simply thoughtless act. In some cases children stumble upon information about the behavior by reading about it in a newspaper or on the internet, or even seeing it on television.

3. **Safety**

   It is always the responsibility of adults to protect the interests and welfare of children. While every child needs to be educated on how to protect him- or herself and what to do in the case of suspected or known molestation behavior, this discussion is even more warranted when you believe your partner has an orientation toward children. But do not automatically equate sex addiction with child molestation. The word addiction can mislead some people to believe that this person has no control over any aspect of his sexuality. That is not true. Addicts tend to act out in ways that are directly related to their own childhood wounding.

If your partner has been engaged in child pornography or known to sexually act out with minors, your children are at risk, and this warrants asking your children whether or not they have ever been inappropriately asked to do something sexual for or with your partner. But I say this with caution. It is very easy to take your outrage and fear and distort the situation. I strongly suggest you allow a qualified helping professional to assist you with this discussion, including the words to use and the timing. This professional needs to be associated with a reputable, licensed agency to ensure that he or she will be able to respond to the needs of the children.

If your children are at risk, then it is appropriate for limits to be set in place that preclude the addict from being with the children or having supervision when they are together. These boundaries remain in place and are renegotiated with suggested oversight of a professional. At this stage, state, social, and health services and courts are often involved and will be making the decisions about parental access to the children.

4. **Breaking the Generational Cycle**
   An age-appropriate, open, honest discussion and education on the basics of addiction and recovery will help you end the generational repetition that occurs in addictive family

systems. Addiction thrives in secrecy so it is important to model healthy sharing of information in your family. You are showing your children that when something happens and you are scared, ashamed, and confused, the best thing to do is talk about it. When openly discussed, almost any problem can be solved. A healthy discussion conveys the message that "In this family we can talk about the hard stuff, and you will be supported and heard."

Appropriate Age

At what age is disclosure most appropriate? My judgment is that a minimum age of mid-adolescence is advised. Children who are pre- or early adolescent should only be told in situations where the children's safety is at risk or their exposure to the information via another avenue, such as at school, from a sibling, or from the media, is possible. Even though the pre- and early adolescents in our research said they were aware of their parent's acting-out behavior, developmentally their greatest need is a belief in the stability of their family. It is the children's own sense of security that is most challenged at this moment. To have sexual data about their parent prior to mid-adolescence is too confusing for them to be able to derive positive meaning or value from having that information. Certainly, maturity of children varies greatly so the professional involved in your situation needs to individually assess the maturity level of your children. By mid-adolescence, as much as children don't want to be told, the information will validate their perceptions and help them better cope with the family stress.

There are times when your preadolescent children's behavior may be the greatest indicator of the need to disclose. They may be acting out confusion, fear, or anger in aggressive or otherwise destructive ways; or they may demonstrate sexual behavior premature to their development (a nine-year-old hiding pornographic pictures, for example). They may repeatedly ask questions that point to some knowledge on their part (such as "Is Dad working late with that woman again?"). You may see their grades slip. They may revert to bedwetting. They may become socially withdrawn or clingy. Due to the many variables of the family system, the individual children, and the extent and type of sexual behavior acted out, determination about disclosure for pre- and mid-adolescent children must be made on a case-by-case basis.

Healthy Disclosure

It is likely that your opportunity to tell your children about what's been going on will present itself in a less than ideal setting, but by being prepared you can still make the most of the opportunity. Following these criteria will make your disclosure a healthier experience for the children:

- Disclosure is best facilitated with a clinician or therapist.

- Both parents should be present and participatory.

- Both parents should be in agreement to disclose to the children.

- Both parents should strategize and agree upon what is and is not disclosed.

- Both parents should speak for themselves about their own behavior.

- Both parents should speak in generalities, not specific details.

- Both parents should display signs of recovery.

- Neither parent should take on the role of victim.

- Children should not be used as confidants by parent(s).

- Both parents should be clear that it is not the children's responsibility to fix or take care of their parents' needs. It is very easy for the children to become caught in a triangle of choosing sides and then reacting on behalf of the person who is perceived to be the victim-parent at the moment.

- Both parents should demonstrate an ongoing openness for dialogue and discussion with a clinician.

- Both parents should make sure the children know they can have further discussions whenever they need to. To say or imply, "We'll talk about this today and never again talk about it" reinforces the shame of disclosure and the behavior. Disclosure is not a one-time discussion.

- The children should be offered the opportunity to talk to a counselor or therapist.

Talking to children about the real issues is a much more difficult conversation if the addicted person is continuing to act out or the two of you are simply not in agreement as to what and when to share. Before you disclose to your children, talk to other women in recovery or a skilled therapist; their experience may prove very helpful as you sort through your specific situation. Even if it becomes essential to talk to your children by yourself, be sure to follow the guidelines discussed in these pages, under Rationale for Disclosure to Children and Appropriate Age, and to seriously consider your motivation.

As a parent, always follow this basic rule: Exercise caution whenever you intend to disclose sensitive information to children. Always consider what is best for the children. It is the responsibility of parents and helping professionals to reassure children that the adults are handling things and taking control of this painful situation.

Whether or not the children ask directly, there are crucial concerns that need to be addressed during the disclosure. The words addiction and compulsivity don't make sense to most children. Describe behaviors such as having secrets, lying, or being unfaithful in an age appropriate language.

If the children are adolescents or older it can be helpful to convey how the parent's behavior was about gaining control and power to overcome feelings of powerlessness, responding to unhealthy anger, medicating and anesthetizing pain, or bolstering self-esteem, and these became more important than anything else. That is the nature of addiction.

Acknowledge how both parents' behaviors have impacted the family as it pertains directly to the children. Will the children be affected by financial consequences, the possibility of marital separation or divorce, changing of schools and losing friendships, or possibly public exposure?

For example, you may find yourself saying, "As a consequence of the behavior . . .

- . . . I wasn't spending time with you; when I was home, I was preoccupied."

- . . . when I was angry with your father I often took my anger out on you."

- . . . I spent what was family money on nonfamily activities."

- . . . there are legal problems that are public and will create embarrassment for the family."

- . . . I have not been available to model healthy relationship behavior."

Again, it is best for each parent to speak for him- or herself and use language that is age-appropriate.

When children ask for specific details such as who, where, and when, it is advised you tell them that this information has been shared only with their other parent unless the answer has a direct impact on them (the children). An example of such a situation needing greater detail might be when a family needs to move or not see a certain relative on a holiday.

I know you may be gasping as you read this. This is a difficult situation, but keeping the following key questions in mind will help guide you. Remember, age is a significant gauge. Ask yourself:

- What is in the best interest of the children?

- How is it helpful for the children to have this knowledge?

- How will it be hurtful for the children not to know?

A SOFT APPROACH TO DISCLOSURE

The following couple took a less direct or what is thought of as a soft approach to disclosure. They recognized the value of sharing but delayed sharing the sexual component for a few years. Should you choose the softer style, you have the option of sharing the message when you believe your child is more developmentally prepared.

[PARTNER]

My kids were seven and nine when everything came out in the open. They had seen and heard anger and crying, and they were aware their father had been absent a lot. When my husband went to treatment and I started my therapy, we simply told the kids that we had done some things to each other that were hurtful; that we had not been honest with each other and now we were working on that. I thought the best thing I could do for them was to keep a routine to their lives. I used my dear friends for backup, people the kids knew and trusted, during these initial treatment experiences. Their father and I told them that we loved them, that these problems were not about them, and that we were going to try very hard to work things out and have a happy family.

While you may choose not to share information with your kids about the sexual aspect of your partner's acting out, their experiences related to the stress within the family need to be validated and they need to be supported. Children of all ages witness tears and anger, and they pick up on the stress between their parents. Basic information can easily validate their perceptions: "Your dad and I are sad right now about how we have treated each other. We are working on being kind to each other. There have been lies and secrets and now we are being honest with each other. We love you and we are sorry we have not paid attention to you and that we have lashed out at you when we were angry with each other. Yes, we are having some adult problems, but they are not about you. You are precious to us and we both love you very much."

In hindsight, the parents in the next two situations wish they had taken a softer approach to disclosure.

[ADDICT]

Looking back I think my children, who were under twelve, were too young to hear so much about my behavior. I don't think they really understood other than their father had done some really bad things that were causing a lot of anger and anguish. I think their being exposed to the information has influenced their dating relationships. But it is also hard to separate how much they were influenced by the dysfunction of my sex addiction and/or the hostile relationship their mother and I were openly engaged in for a lot of their early lives.

Because they had heard and seen so much, they needed to be told something. But it wasn't like a private discussion with the focus being what was best for them. We should have been coached in how to think like that. Or until we could be more civil with each other, it should have been left with saying their parents had some problems and were angry with each other but that we were trying to work it out. Then our efforts should have been in getting into some healthy family routines.

[JENNY]

As I look back, our kids were ten, sixteen, seventeen, and nineteen. In the moment it seemed so appropriate to get all the secrets out. In hindsight, I think their father and I should have dealt with how our behavior had affected the kids' lives, made amends to them, told them we were getting help, and then delayed the disclosure of the sex addiction until we had experienced some healing and stabilized the environment. I can see the risk in this too; the environment may never stabilize. Nonetheless, I do think there is a time and place for disclosing the secrets. We could have been more general in sharing with them early on and dealt with the specifics later.

A DIRECT APPROACH TO DISCLOSURE

The following are two examples of couples who chose a very direct style of disclosure and felt good about this approach in their family.

[PARTNER]

My husband and I together told our nineteen- and twenty-one-year-old sons only after their father went to treatment. They thought he was in treatment for using pills. And he was. But we knew he was there for sex, too. We didn't tell them a lot in the disclosure to them. But we told them that he had been having affairs throughout our marriage, and we wanted them to know because we didn't want any more family secrets. We both think they knew he had affairs, and it was important to us that they heard that there is an addiction component to this behavior. We felt it was our responsibility to educate. My husband did most of the talking. He and I had agreed to that so they could hear it from him, and not me who had been this angry wife/mother for so long. We thought they would just think it was me being punishing. They didn't ask much. They wanted to know if the last affair was really over. They wanted to know if we were considering a divorce. Later, when our younger son was twenty-three, he came to my husband and said he needed help for his sex addiction. He actually used those words. He was acting out on the internet. Had we not been honest and had we not made the changes we made in our recovery, I don't know if he would have come to his father for help.

[MAITE]

My children, both young teenagers, know almost everything except some matters that involve legal issues. Both of us shared with them when they asked questions as to why we went to recovery meetings. We explained to them that we as husband and wife have problems and we need to heal. And the way to heal is to commit seriously to changing how we relate to each other. If not, we will be too sick to be a good mom and dad.

These parents shared to validate the children's experience; they shared to stop the secret keeping; and they shared in hope that it would help prevent the dysfunction in their family from repeating generationally.

RECOGNIZING THE COMPLEXITY

No doubt this is difficult. The following example shares the complexity of parents doing what they think is the right thing, recognizing how traumatic the information can be and second-guessing their decision. Ultimately, several years later, they are grateful for the recovery the family as a whole has been able to experience.

[PARTNER]

What I remember is my husband and I telling our nine- and eleven-year-old kids. Over the next few weeks and months, our nine-year-old daughter started to wet her bed at night. She was crying a lot. Looking back I see how very traumatic it was. One night, nine years later, we were watching a movie that reminded her of our family back then and she suddenly started to cry. She cried like a baby in my arms and told me she shouldn't have been told so much about our problems. That is true, she shouldn't have, but I also know she shouldn't have had to be with parents who were so unhealthy, who were so dysfunctional in their lives. When I think about the overall big picture, the outcome is good. She and her brother would not only witness our "War of the Roses" years and our struggles in early recovery, but would ultimately come to see us committed to our recovery practices, committed to our family, and living in the truth.

Clearly, the decisions around disclosure are hard to make. Would I have done it differently? I really don't know, given that our family is in good shape today. I only know my experience. It is hard to know how best to do it.

For some parent(s) what you share and when is obvious, but as you can see, for others it is not so apparent. What complicates the situation is that often you are making an initial decision very early in your own recovery process and, in many cases, attempting to make this decision with a partner who is looking at this situation through different eyes. While age and timing are significant, the setting and how to answer their concerns are important considerations for this to be a constructive experience.

ANSWERING THEIR QUESTIONS

The following is a list of questions children may pose to you during disclosure. Rehearsing how you would answer such questions will make the conversation go smoother.

Do you still love each other?

Children want to know how parents feel about each other. This may be a difficult question to answer. Your answer may be a resounding yes. If this is not the reality, you might say, "I am very angry, and I'm questioning how I feel." Or you may only be able to say, "I don't know, I am sorting it out." But that needs to be followed with reassurance that this does not affect how much you love them.

Did I do something wrong?

Children need to hear that what is happening between their parents is not about them or their behavior, but about the parents' relationship. Young and adolescent children are very quick to think they are responsible for others' behaviors and feelings. It is critical you are clear this is a problem between you and your partner, not about them.

How does this affect my life?

A child's greatest concern is usually whether or not his or her parents will remain together. If as a parent you are not sure what may happen for your family, you can express your uncertainty and then commit to tell the children when you do know. But often what they are also asking or wanting to ask is more immediate and more specific to their day, such as, "Will you be at my play performance next week?" "What about our vacation we were going on in two months?" "Will there be enough money for me to go to camp?" "To school?" "How does this impact my birthday?" Reassure them of their knowing about any change in routine and encourage them to ask such questions if they are concerned.

Who else knows?

It is important to discuss who else knows. The disclosure itself should not become the family secret. Recovery is not about replacing one secret with another. Recovery is demonstrating healthy boundaries and being discriminating with whom one does and does not share. If other people know, prepare your children with an honest response to the questions and remarks of others.

Are you sorry?

Children need to hear and consequently come to believe that both of their parents are sorry for their hurtful behavior. Children need to know you are sorry and see you making whatever behavior amends you can. Making amends takes time. Time and healthy new behaviors allow the possibility of genuine forgiveness to occur. It is not appropriate to ask your children to forgive you. Remember, this conversation is really about what is best for them, not about shifting the focus onto you.

What is happening so that things will get better?

Children need to be told about your recovery plans. If possible they need to know what both adults are doing to help the relationship and the family. You may only be able to speak to the immediate, but they need a sense of security that there is a plan so things could get better.

As you consider whether to disclose your situation to your children, you may also find it helpful to hear what some children thought would have improved their disclosure experiences.

"A little humility would have made me feel better about my dad."

"Dad really let Mom do most of the talking. I would have preferred he said more."

"Not so much detail."

"My stepmom went crazy. She shouldn't have been so angry in front of us."

"More resources like reading material about sex addiction."

"Questions should be accepted, even welcomed, so the family unit can face the problem in its entirety."

"A qualified therapist present would make the disclosure much easier."

"A counselor who didn't just work with my dad would have been better."

"I should have been taken to counseling again when I got a couple years older."

ONGOING HEALING

Discussing the situation will undoubtedly elicit a multitude of feelings for every family member. At the time of the sharing and after, parents and clinicians need to be willing and available to listen and validate the children's feelings. This may be very painful for parents but it is a necessary part of healing for the family. As an adult child responded in her questionnaire:

"Truth, even if in very small pieces, can lighten
the load. Shame is a burden we as children should
not have to bear."

Of course you do not want to cause your children pain, but
that ideal is lost in the act of the addiction. Parents must forgive
themselves for their behavior, move on in recovery, and learn
recovery skills. Those skills begin with honesty to yourself and
then to appropriate others.

You may be wondering how much you should update your
children during the recovery process.

[SARA]

Several years after an initial disclosure, my
husband's acting out worsened and we didn't tell
our children. They didn't need to know the ups and
downs of our marriage. But when the day came
that we decided we needed a separation, we told
our three children, now aged nineteen to twenty-
five, of their father's escalating sexual behavior
and that together we had made the decision to
have a therapeutic separation. Then we explained
what that meant. In this process, knowing that two
of our children were struggling with committed
relationships, I decided it was time I shared a
secret only my husband knew: that a few years
back, in my anger, I had an affair. My rationale in
telling them was that it was time for the family
secrets to end and to help my kids see how people
do hurtful things when they are angry. I didn't
expect or ask for understanding or forgiveness; I
just needed honesty. Our kids struggled with their
own immediate anger, fear, and sadness. But ours
was a family wherein the parenting from both my
husband and me was strong. All three kids, without

offering resistance, accepted what we needed to do
to help our marriage.

Your children of any age do not need to be kept abreast of the day-to-day progress of either your or your partner's recovery. They need to be allowed to focus on what is most relevant to their lives (such as school, friends, work, or newly created families or careers). Regardless of age, they need and desire your well-being. Their lives are more secure knowing their parents are attending to their recovery practices. Teens and older children can make sense of the overall picture, but giving them details of the addicted parent's triggers or relapses (unless that information has a direct impact on their lives) violates a healthy parent–child boundary.

Beyond Disclosure

Stopping the possibility of a generational legacy involves more than a candid conversation. It really begins with your recovery as parents. Whether or not they are aware of the sexual acting out, children are much more impacted by the family dynamics. Your children's relationship with the addict may be emotionally distressed as a consequence of his physical absences, his not showing up to events, his lies and broken promises, or his emotional absence or overindulgence at home. Rageful behavior and mismanagement of money create consequences for children; but this isn't just about the addict's behavior. If the two of you demonstrate poor relational skills such as anger, silence, sarcasm, or inattentiveness, then that is also problematic. Your behavior has a direct impact on your children as well. Distorted anger, depression, using your kids to communicate for you, not allowing them their autonomy, or using them as your confidant or friend are just a few of the ways your behavior could also fuel long-term problems. The direct pain children experience is just as often about the unhealthy expression of emotions and poor relational skills as it may be about sexual messages and behavior.

History has proven that time and time again, in the throes of living with addictive behavior, whether or not it is recognized as such, children experience emotional abandonment that sets them up to seek ways to escape or numb their pain, often leading to various forms of addiction.

Children growing up with addiction often vow, "It will never happen to me." Yet when they meet with life's difficulties, they don't have the emotional maturity or coping skills to live their life differently. Historically, when young people are hurt, confused, and angry, they resort to acting out with alcohol, other drugs, and/or sex. They begin to repeat the models they were raised with, all the while rationalizing, minimizing, and denying that they too are a part of the addictive cycle. They act out sexually or, as the Women of the Lodge said, "become the perfect partner."

My intent here is not to scare you, but to help you garner a healthy fear of the insidiousness of the generational repetition of addiction—repetition that is only broken by way of a recovery process. There is a saying, "When addiction exists within a family, look a second time." I would like to rephrase that slightly as "When recovery exists in a family, look again." You have the potential to stop the legacy of addiction and sexual betrayal and significantly improve the odds that healthy choices and lifestyle come naturally in your children's development.

More so than words, your style of parenting will have the greatest impact in the long run. Take responsibility where you can. The resiliency of children will be supported when you:

- Keep your children's lives on track.

- Maintain healthy family rituals and traditions.

- Listen attentively.

- Develop healthy boundaries.

- Validate emotions.

- Model and teach problem-solving skills.

- Model healthy ways of coping with stress.

- Protect your children as appropriate.

- Steer your children toward appropriate resources.

- Realize the relationship your children have with their other parent is theirs and not yours

- Engage in your own recovery practices

You cannot change the past behavior, but you can influence your children by providing an example in your recovery practices. If you do not have a commitment to change your family system, disclosure alone won't break this addiction cycle. Changing the family system begins with your individual commitment to recovery. Then, at the appropriate time, disclosing secrets to your children can help to break the generational cycle.

It is in recovery that you will find the strength to be the parent your children need you to be. You will probably always feel sad that your children have been exposed to dynamics that have caused them pain. It is normal to be concerned and fearful of the consequences for your children. With support from others in recovery and with the guidance of skilled helping professionals, you can do your part by taking responsibility and being accountable to your children.

Reflective Thoughts and Questions

- What are your concerns about your children?

- What are your thoughts about whether or not you will disclose your situation to your children and help them move into healing?

- Identify skills and practices you and your partner do that you believe contribute to healthy parenting.

- Identify behaviors and practices you and your partner do that you believe are detrimental to healthy parenting.

- Identify three behaviors you believe will strengthen healthy parenting.

- What was important for you to learn in this chapter?

CHAPTER SIX NOTES

1   Claudia Black, Diane Dillon, and Stefanie Carnes, "Disclosure to Children: Hearing the Child's Experience," *Sexual Addiction & Compulsivity* 10, no. 1 (2003): 67–78.

CHAPTER SEVEN

Your Time to Heal

How long will it hurt?

Will I ever be able to trust again?

Is there help?

Your recovery will not be linear; there will be no straight lines. Some women describe it as a crazed meandering journey through dense clouds.

Undoubtedly it is arduous; there will be many ups and downs. You cannot schedule it; there is no timetable for any leg of your journey. It is an expanding process that begins with willingness, from a place of pain (and sometimes relief), and it unfolds differently for everyone. To begin your healing—your recovery journey—you must stop pretending, denying, minimizing, and rationalizing. You may come to recovery angry, defeated, embarrassed, ashamed, or confused, but just come. Remember the wonderful saying, "When you are at the end of your rope, let go." You have held on so long that your arms are tired, your muscles have been stretched and pulled, and your hands are raw.

You may feel that if you let go, you will fall. But the Women of the Lodge discovered that it was "hanging on" that caused their pain.

When the chat rooms were not enough, he went to strip shows; when they weren't enough, he bought the girls and took them back to his hotel room. It didn't matter how many of them he had; it was never enough. Now I have had enough. Enough hurting, enough crying, enough bargaining; it is my time to heal.

Boundaries, Boundaries, Boundaries

No boundaries, walled boundaries, damaged boundaries—everything but healthy boundaries. Boundary violation and distortion is a given at such times of crisis. When you live with boundary violation and distortion, it erodes your esteem and creates confusion about who is responsible for what. You lose the ability to maintain what is called "protection" boundaries and often react without "containment" boundaries. Not having the knowledge of what is occurring, being gaslighted, and succumbing to the manipulations, sets you up for becoming a victim and/or victimizing others. Both are common responses to being traumatized. Living with an addict only reinforces boundary violations because addicts are masters at trampling on boundaries. In time, as your esteem is battered, your boundaries sustain major damage. Your greatest source of strength and safety will come from self-care and that includes the use of effective boundaries.

[JACQUE]

I had heard that word "boundaries," but in reality it meant nothing to me, as I had so few. I let myself be talked into doing things I didn't want to do sexually. I allowed myself to sit and listen to him tell me everything that was wrong with me. I was truly a doormat. I felt so poorly about myself that I just wouldn't stand up for myself with any self-respect.

Developing boundaries means knowing your physical and psychological comfort zone—your safety zone—and knowing what you like and don't like. It is having a sense of your own self, separate from others. It defines you as a separate human being, not someone else's possession. Your ability to protect yourself psychologically and physically is linked to the durability of your boundaries. The skill to develop healthy boundaries is limit setting. They are mechanisms that bring safety into your life by establishing healthy control. As you strengthen your boundaries you gain a clearer sense of control of yourself and your relationship with others; they empower you to determine how you'll be treated by others. Boundaries are statements about what you will and will not do, acting as limits for what others can and cannot do to you. By setting boundaries for yourself, you are exercising your inherent power to declare that you are a separate and independent individual, not a possession or extension of anyone else. This skill is vital to defining who you are and how you will be treated.

You don't set boundaries to punish another person; you set them to honor and protect yourself. It is up to you to decide how you want to live and what you can and cannot live with. It is up to you to set boundaries that help you feel safe and confident so you can heal. This takes time, but you can do it.

While people readily recognize physical boundaries, we also have emotional, sexual, relational, intellectual, financial, and spiritual boundaries. Emotional boundaries define the self: our ideas, feelings, and values. We set emotional boundaries by choosing how we let people treat us. Our spiritual development comes from our inner self. Only we know the spiritual path for ourselves. We have sexual boundaries: limits on what is safe and appropriate sexual behavior. We have a choice about who we interact with sexually and the extent of that interaction. We have relationship boundaries. These boundaries define the limits and expansion of appropriate interaction with others. Our intellectual boundaries offer us the opportunity to enjoy learning and teaching. They allow us to be curious and inspired.

It's important to establish boundaries that are flexible but within limits; they can shift appropriately in response to situations: out for strangers, in for those you are intimate with; out for those you don't feel safe with, in for those you trust. For example, you may not find it acceptable for a stranger to give you a hug, but you are willing to receive a hug from a family member. It is not okay for an acquaintance to expect to stay at your house while on vacation, but that might be an appropriate expectation from friends or family members. Boundaries should be fixed enough to preserve your individual self, yet open to considering new ideas. They are firm enough to uphold values and priorities, and open enough to communicate your priorities. Having healthy boundaries convey that you have determined certain behaviors are inappropriate and/or appropriate in the context of certain relationships. As a consequence, emotional, physical, sexual, spiritual, and financial safety can be created by the use of effective boundaries.

Living a life of intimidation, doubting your own perceptions, partners find it almost impossible to protect or defend themselves when it might upset the addict. Your response is to back off; to retreat. In recovery, you need to learn to strike a balance between showing respect and concern for others and equally showing respect and concern for yourself; not reacting from a place of fear but inner strength.

[PARTNER]

I was so afraid to say that I needed things to be a certain way for me in this relationship. He started attending these groups, but I just wanted him to tell me what he was going to do differently. I wanted him to be different because I didn't know if I could really live and be on my own. I had two kids and there was no child support from their father. But I listened to other women start to say it was important for me to respect myself and not to stay in my fear. So little by little I started to say what I thought and what I felt, and then the biggie—what I needed. With that, I was setting boundaries.

When partners are being harmed or attacked, they tend to want to analyze the situation rather than take cover. Let me share with you a riddle that stumps many people: "If you are standing under a window and someone starts dumping garbage on top of your head, what do you do?"

Long pause.

Then the woman replies tentatively, "Ask them to stop?"

The answer and the appropriate response is, "You get out of the way. You move."

This isn't the moment to ask why; it's the time to take care of yourself. While a lack of boundaries sets you up for being a victim, it can also set you up to be hurtful and intrusive to others. Going in either direction is an act of being boundary-less. You are not protecting yourself when you are in a victim stance. You also demonstrate a lack of boundaries when you fail to respect the boundaries of others. Healthy boundaries reinforce your inner worth and value, and support your integrity and self-worth.

[SARA]

A lot of my problems with boundaries had to do with my being uncontained. I'd flip from totally walled boundaries to being boundary-less. And when I did, I was hurtful to others. I had this wall of silence where I literally said nothing. When I finally spoke up to my husband, I preached and ranted! Certainly his behavior toward me was abusive, but I was abusive too, in other ways. And then having no boundaries, it was like I was leaking all over. I was telling everyone what was going on with him and others. I called his family and told them. I told his coworkers. I even told the hairdresser, who didn't know either of us. I was telling anybody and everybody.

Maintaining boundaries that prevent you from being retaliatory can sometimes be challenging. Yes, you have the right to be angry, even outraged, but being boundary-less only inflames greater chaos and drama.

SAYING NO, SAYING YES

Boundaries enable you to embrace both the words *no* and *yes*. While the words are not usually verbalized within boundaries, they are the underpinnings. When being belittled, harshly criticized, or being raged at, to say nothing or to remain in the situation is in essence saying, "Yes, I deserve this" or "Yes, I am helpless and must endure." Saying no to this behavior is saying, "Stop, you are disrespecting me" or "I will listen to you when you speak more respectfully to me, but not now." And if he doesn't stop, say, "I am willing to talk about whatever it is you are angry about at another time when you can speak to me differently. Right now I am going in the other room and you are not to follow me." By saying, "No, this behavior is disrespectful," you are saying yes to yourself.

If you are out to dinner with your partner and you perceive him being preoccupied with other women in the restaurant, setting a boundary in which you honor yourself would be saying no to the situation. You would also be saying yes to yourself by telling him something such as, "I am uncomfortable with you starting conversations with the other women at the tables, please refrain from looking in their direction and engaging in conversation with them."

If your relationship with the addict is one where he controls the money, and you want to say no to this dynamic and yes to honoring yourself with a more mutual relationship around money, your boundary may be when you say something such as, "I need to have my name on all of our bank accounts and on our stock portfolios." On the flip side, if you are lacking containment and you find yourself raging at someone, you rein in your boundary-less behavior by saying no to yourself: "No, I am not entitled to be abusive toward him," and "Yes, I will honor my self-respect and find another way in which to tell him what I am thinking and feeling."

In your healing, explore what the words *no* and *yes* have meant to you. Consider how your inability to say no or yes have been hurtful to you. Challenge your beliefs about the meanings that might underlie these words. Does saying no mean you won't be liked? Does it mean you aren't a nice person? Does it mean people will avoid you? Does saying yes prevent you from being rejected? Does saying yes make you feel lovable? Does saying yes help you avoid uncomfortable feelings? While the words *no* and *yes* are small in size, in recovery they are powerful and are crucial to having healthy boundaries.

Early Recovery Boundaries

In early recovery the boundaries you set around the addict's behavior will help stabilize your situation. These boundaries state what you need to do for your own integrity and self-respect. To this you will have to say what is not acceptable behavior on the addict's part. You have probably already begun to discern what you deem to be unacceptable behavior. Now it's time to communicate those healthy boundaries. By failing to do so—not owning your reality, your truth—you are treating yourself with the same disregard your partner has shown you.

The following will give you an idea of different boundaries other partners have established for themselves.

- I will not engage in sex acts I find demeaning, repugnant, or uncomfortable.

- When my husband makes sexual remarks under the guise of humor, I will tell him I find that behavior offensive.

- I will not engage with him sexually until we both have been tested for sexually transmitted diseases.

- It is not okay with me for him to take women to lunch alone, business or personal. I will request that of him.

Note that these boundaries are about what you will do, not what you are insisting he do. You only have the power to request, to take action for yourself; you cannot make him do something.

Other boundaries you may make are ones such as:

- You decide with whom and how much to share about your situation with others.

- You will ask your partner to do certain things that give you a greater sense of safety such as putting a filter on electronic devices or putting your name on certain legal documents.

- Common boundaries are those established around what type of touch is okay—a hug, a kiss on the cheek or lips.

- Taking a time out when in a conversation and you feel as if you cannot maintain your protection or containment boundaries.

Nonnegotiable Boundaries

It is also common to have what are referred to as nonnegotiable boundaries. This is a boundary involving something you must have or something you can't tolerate in order to stay in a relationship. They are relationship deal breakers. Therefore you need to be very careful in stating them. It is strongly suggested that you discuss your desires with a therapist and then when nonnegotiable boundaries are shared with your partner that discussion also occurs with the facilitation of a therapist.

While you may have many boundaries and you may have many requests, for most people there are usually only two or three nonnegotiable boundaries.

Know your nonnegotiable boundaries are specific and unique to your situation. No one can or should tell you what your boundaries must be. The following are examples of nonnegotiable boundaries established by other partners:

- You must stay in your aftercare for at least one year.

- You will have no work-related travel for the next six months.

- You will wear your wedding ring at all times.

- The computer will be in the living room only and will have filters on it.

As you can see, there are time frames for two of the above nonnegotiable boundaries. All four examples are boundaries that can be renegotiated at a later time. These nonnegotiable boundaries are being set to provide greater stability when in crisis.

But when it comes to nonnegotiable, ask yourself, "What would absolutely without question cause me to know I can no longer stay in this relationship?"

Just as you have laid out your nonnegotiable points, the addict is entitled to have some boundaries, and some being nonnegotiable as well.

Examples of his nonnegotiable boundaries might be:

- It is *never* okay to hit me.

- It is not okay to threaten to take the kids away from me.

- You must attend therapy at least once a week.

These boundaries are emotionally laden and are best worked out with a counselor. Honor them as a commitment to your recovery.

If your partner is not pursuing recovery, you will want to strategize how you will present these limits to him. It can be helpful to rehearse this conversation ahead of time so you are more confident. And again, seriously consider having a conversation with a therapist for greater clarity and support.

Setting boundaries means taking responsibility for yourself and reclaiming the power you have given away. It is letting others know what is acceptable to you and what is not. Learning about boundaries takes time. Be patient. Get feedback from other recovering partners and/or a counselor. They will have a perspective you may not have.

Freeing Yourself from the Mental Frenzy

One of the biggest challenges partners face is preoccupation and ruminating thoughts. *Ruminating* is a cognitive attempt to control the situation and/or to avoid the overwhelming emotions of the situation at a time when you are trying to make sense of it. "If I can picture it, I can figure it out." "If I can say the right thing, I'll stop his behavior/punish him/hurt him." This mental vigilance is a form of traumatizing yourself. You can be so consumed in your mind-set of preoccupation and rumination that it feels as if you are going crazy with the various images. To get out of your head means getting in touch with the feelings you are carrying. Freeing yourself from that state requires a willingness to begin to show and share those feelings, recognizing that you are the one keeping yourself trapped in this mental frenzy. It begins by accepting that preoccupation doesn't help your situation and only keeps you trapped in defeated thinking.

Let me share with you how some of the Women of the Lodge addressed this.

[JACQUE]

I journal because I need to get it out of my head. Putting my thoughts and feelings down on paper has been a great tool for me. I catch myself and STOP—STOP—STOP. I see this as my scared little girl inside of me, and I speak to her. I thank her for sharing, for telling me how scared she is, but I tell her that I am doing well now and can take care of myself in a way I haven't been able to before. It's like setting limits with your child. I set limits with myself. I just stop. Sometimes it just does not work, so then I call another woman in my group and tell her I am struggling.

[MAITE]

I use the Serenity Prayer.[1] Over and over and over. Today it truly is not a problem for me.

[SARA]

Oh, this has been a big one. I can get going in my head and that takes on a life of its own. One time on our way to the airport to take a trip, I had been thinking about things and suddenly I insisted he give me some details about what he did when he was with this last woman. I got focused on the sex act itself. Well, he refused to be specific. I got more and more mad, furious. By the time we arrived at the airport I refused to go on the trip, threw him his suitcase, and raced away in our car. He got on the plane and called me later. I was sure he would apologize. He called to let me know that I had thrown my own suitcase at him and he had my things. Today when I start down that road of ruminating and obsessing, I just say, "Take a hammer and hit yourself on the head because the only person you are harming is you."

As Sara said, "This has been a big one." Obsession and ruminating are major challenges. I don't know that I've ever worked with a partner who didn't struggle with obsessive thoughts. Vanessa found some answers in the use of a practice she called the God Box.

[VANESSA]

I use my God Box. I pray. Left to my own devices I will only ruminate and obsess. I was introduced to this concept by other recovering women who told me that they keep an actual box for this purpose. Mine sits on a shelf. So when I get into my fear and realize it, I put it down on paper and say this, "I turn it over to you." And sometime during the day I will make sure it gets to the God Box.

Many women in recovery use a God Box; others refer to this as their Worry Box. It can be as simple as a shoebox or as fancy as a specially chosen decorative box. It's designated as the repository for those thoughts you know you can no longer carry and still maintain your health. You simply write down your thoughts and put them in the God Box. In this way, you turn your worry over to your Higher Power.

Ruminating and preoccupation are both understandable and yet immobilizing. As natural as this behavior is, remember you are only hurting yourself with it. It is as if you are drinking poison and hoping the other person will die. When you find yourself ruminating or projecting, ask yourself, "What can I do about this right now? Is there action I can take? A decision I can make? Something tangible I can accomplish at the moment?" If so, do it. If not, let the problem go for the moment. You can do that with the help of prayer, deep breathing, meditation, and support. Keep your head where your feet are—together in the present. Then get focused on other aspects of your life. Get ready for work, make needed appointments, exercise, or finish a project. With specific recovery practices and support, you can quiet your obsessive thinking.

Calming the Emotional Brain

It's an understatement that this has been a painful journey. But as with any trauma and its consequences, it does not need to be a life sentence. No matter how deep or painful your trauma may be, healing is possible. I know this because I have seen it many times. This healing begins with inner stability. You need to find ways to soothe yourself and feel safe in your own skin. Grounding practices help you to manage your feelings, both when you experience pain in the present and when you examine painful events of the past. They are not rocket science, they are learnable, tried-and-true tools to help your nervous system regulate and limbic system become calm. You may already practice some of them. Many are fun, pleasurable, and most are free or inexpensive. They are not meant to be used once or twice, but are to be regular practices you integrate into your life.

Common forms of grounding include:

- Writing to include journaling, creative writing, poetry, etc.

- Gardening.

- Time in nature.

- Mindfulness practices, most commonly forms of meditation and mindful walking.

- Crafting, be it needlepoint, woodworking, bead making, quilting, paper making, etc.

- Knitting, crocheting.

- Creating art, via painting, sculpting, drawing, photography, etc.

- Engagement with animals, equine (horse) therapy.

- Dancing.

- Singing.

- Martial arts.

- Tai chi.

- Yoga.

Given what has been occurring in your life I can only imagine what you are thinking. "When is there time for me to do these things? I have way too many serious things going on. My life is falling apart." Yet there is science behind many of these practices demonstrating their value to people who have experienced trauma. They can:

- Improve memory.

- Calm a racing mind or obsessive thoughts.

- Reduce stress.

- Improve attention, focus, and ability to concentrate.

- Reduce depression.

- Make it easier to interrupt patterns of addiction.

- Reduce emotional reactivity and over-the-top responses.

- Make sleep easier to fall into, deeper, and more refreshing.

- Increase compassion for yourself and others.

All of these benefits speak to the needs of partners. Begin by just choosing a couple and integrate them into your daily life.

Concept of Powerlessness

The confusion and pain you experience due to the addict's behavior lead you to become increasingly focused on your partner. You have been fighting a demon in the coupleship that was often unnamed and would go in and out of visibility. You have been doing what you can to make your relationship work. The betrayal is eating away at your heart and soul and you are doing what you can to fight the beast. Yet in this process, you may fail to recognize how some of your own behavior creates chaos and is hurtful in your life.

The addict is often referred to a self-help twelve-step program for their sex addiction. Many partners find validation and direction in the twelve-step groups of Recovering Couples Anonymous (RCA) and Co-Sex Addicts Anonymous (COSA). In the twelve-step program, the first step is admitting your powerlessness over the compulsive sexual behavior and recognizing how your life has become unmanageable as a consequence of your own behavior. This is not to dismiss what has happened to you. This is to help you become aware of your own self-defeating behavior in reaction to this trauma and in the process help you identify what behaviors you can let go of that enhance your own well-being. So with compassion for self, be open to identifying any of your behaviors that would lessen your own frenzy.

For the time being, focus on surrendering control of your partner and his behavior. Begin by asking yourself in what ways you try to control him or the situation.

- Do I lie or make excuses for him?

- Do I check through his personal belongings?

- Do I yell? Threaten? Plead? Demand?

- Am I sexual when I don't want to be, in ways I do not want to be?

- Do I throw out his stash or monitor email messages, purchases, or mileage?

- Do I try to avoid social situations in a manner that I think limits his access to the object of his desires?

- Do I give him the silent treatment?

In the long run, have any of these behaviors made a difference? This is a critical question. In the long run it hasn't, it only has driven you further to distraction and been retraumatizing.

Think about how your denial, preoccupation with the addict, lack of self-care, lack of healthy boundaries, and your defenses have contributed to your pain and confusion.

- What toll have these problems taken on you physically? Describe physical symptoms such as loss of sleep, headaches, gastrointestinal problems, back pain, weight gain, or weight loss.

- What effect has there been on your physical appearance? Are you obsessive about your appearance? Do you take less pride in your grooming and dress?

- What effect has there been on you sexually? (Did you have an affair, engage in sex acts that you didn't want to, avoid sex?) Has this behavior affected how you feel as a woman?

- What effect has there been on you emotionally? Are you depressed? Angry all the time? Are you displacing your feelings? Numb?

- What effect has there been on you spiritually? Are you reluctant to seek a spiritual path? If so, what is that reluctance about? Do your religious beliefs interfere with asserting yourself?

- What effect has there been on you intellectually? Do you think you are stupid? Incapable? Forgetful? Preoccupied?

- What effect has there been on your parenting? Are you being overprotective? A super parent? Distancing? Rageful? Inattentive? Neglectful? Too enmeshed?

- What effect has there been on your friendships? Do you find yourself lying or making excuses for your partner's behavior, his absences, his ogling, and his sexualized comments? Are you isolating?

- What effect has there been on your work? Have your attendance and performance been impacted? Are you working overtime? Are you changing jobs frequently?

- What effect is there in the area of responsibility? Are you being overly responsible or irresponsible?

- What effect has there been on your daily routine? Are you "dancing as fast as you can" with busyness? Are you feeling the stress of perfectionism?

These are some of the issues twelve-step programs are referring to when discussing unmanageability. Identifying the unmanageability is about addressing your own self-defeating behavior. It is recognizing what you are powerless over and owning the unmanageability that is related to your own behavior. This is ultimately empowering and can help you move forward in the healing process.

[PARTNER]

I would rehearse what I was going to say to him when he walked through the door, but the minute I saw him all of those thoughts flew out the window and I'd start ranting and raving. There were times I'd be sitting at home imagining what he was doing, making incessant phone calls to locate him. There were nights I'd replay his phone message to me for hours while drinking wine and calling every motel in the city.

[PARTNER]

I was sleep deprived, I was forty pounds overweight, I flipped from crying to rage on a dime, and my husband's latest affair was just exposed on television. A friend suggested that maybe, just maybe, I needed some help. I simply couldn't keep going on pretending while my life was falling apart on every level.

[PARTNER]

He kept asking me to go to the therapist with him, and I was so self-righteous. My husband was so earnest in his recovery. He was like a different person. He was becoming this considerate, accountable man. For three years I hung on to my martyrdom, my anger, my shame. I was becoming more and more cold. It was as if I wanted his old behavior back, the way I egged him on. But he wouldn't engage like the old days, and I saw myself getting sicker and sicker. Thank heaven one day I really was tired of being sick and tired.

As someone who has been traumatized by sexual betrayal, you have the right to want safety, you have the right to want the truth, respect. You do not deserve the shame you feel, and have every reason for your rage, your despair, your confusion. You are on the path. Today in recovery you are more apt to find that safety, self-respect, and to be able to operate from your truth by recognizing where your power lies. With the skills of boundary setting, grounding tools, a framework for knowing what is happening and has happened in your coupleship, you are taking back your life.

Feelings

The challenge with letting go when you're at the end of your rope is that you quickly get in touch with deeper feelings. For some of you the depth of your pain and anguish or fear is so profound that you don't know how you will survive. You remember the images you came across on the computer and how you felt angry and compelled to search for more, all the while thinking your heart was going to break from the despair you felt. These fluctuating emotions often get too scary and the tendency is to avoid them altogether. On the other hand, you may be at the opposite extreme, feeling shut down, numb and frozen, or the flip side so enraged you can't function. Because the trauma is intimate in nature, the emotional work is more challenging as you are vacillating among multitudes of feelings related to the person with whom you may still be in a relationship. It is when you own and accept your feelings—whether you feel angry, fearful, sad, humiliated, or ashamed—that you will be able to embrace life, to move forward. To be whole you need to be able to access a range of feelings. Part of your recovery is learning to identify a wide scope of feelings and then learning the healthy expression of those feelings.

Learning to own your feelings won't be easy because you have probably spent a lifetime not being safe with your feelings. It is likely that you gleaned your understanding of what to do with your feelings from a culture and family that told you which feelings were acceptable and which were not. That modeling then became reinforced in your relationship with someone who sexually acts out. He is not there to listen, to validate, or to offer support. In fact he most often discounts, ignores, and denies your feelings. He rages in anger or walks away in silence. He tells you there is no reason for you to feel the way you do. It's possible he tells you that not only do you have no reason to be fearful, angry, or sad, but in fact you should be grateful.

It is likely you have a lot of fears of what would happen should you show feelings. Fears such as:

- Others won't like me.

- People are going to be able to see how bad I am.

- I'll be seen as weak, and that is bad.

- People will tell me I have no reasons to feel this way.

- I will be out of control, and that is not okay.

- I will be vulnerable to getting hurt.

- People will take advantage of me.

You may be at a stage where you have difficulty expressing your feelings because you have difficulty identifying them. You may not recognize anger as you stand with your fists clenched and arms tightly folded. I have worked with women who had tears rolling down their faces, and when asked what they were feeling, they didn't know. Many women smile broadly through their fear, humiliation, and anger.

Feelings are cues that signal what you need. If you pay attention to your feelings, you will become more adept at knowing your needs. Feelings also help you determine the boundaries you need to set to provide security for yourself. They are your signals to comfort, safety, discomfort, and danger. A mark of recovery is the ability to know what you feel when you feel it—to be comfortable with your emotional self, and then determine whether or not and with whom you share feelings. Feelings are most hurtful to yourself when they are denied, minimized, and when they accumulate. Prior to beginning recovery you may have been avoiding your feelings by eating, shopping, working, exercising, drinking alcohol, or taking other drugs. Maybe you did some sexual acting out yourself. The first step is identifying how you mask your feelings. Then pay attention to when you put that mask on.

In the early stages of healing, your feelings will be all over the map and may seem very contrary to each other. You may feel sad and happy at the same time, or sad and angry, or loving and hateful. This is to be expected. You have not gone crazy. It only means you're sad and happy, sad and angry, or that you love and you hate. It's normal to have multiple and even contrary feelings at the same time.

[MAITE]

Thank heaven I quickly found a women's group with women in similar situations to me. I didn't feel so crazy. My feelings were all over the place. They would flip: in the beginning sometimes from one minute to the next, in time from one hour to the next, then maybe one day to the next. But whatever I was feeling, the other women accepted me. They understood. They laughed with me; they cried with me; they validated my indignation and anger. It was so liberating for me—me who had been Ms. Perfect. Not now, and it is great.

[JENNY]

I didn't think the pain would ever go away. For a long time I was mostly numb. I would see other women in my recovery group so full of feelings. And then I started to thaw. And then feelings began to come: pain, raw pain, anguish, shame, and loneliness. I was so lonely. Fear ran rampant at all times. Then anger. All of this was so new to me.

Like Jenny, sometimes you may wish you could just stay numb. Some partners do just that, but staying numb can lead to depression, forms of self-medication, and even illness. When you stay numb, the hurt continues to grow. Trust that there are reasons for the depth of your feelings. Whatever you feel, it doesn't mean you are a bad person or wrong. What's important is that you are able to talk about those feelings. You don't have to know the sources of your feelings. But you can open your mouth and say, "I'm sad. I don't know what's going on, but I feel sad" or "I'm so angry, I'm angry at everything." The more you verbalize what you do know and what you do feel, the sooner you'll be able to connect your feelings to their origins.

It is usually early in the recovery process that the pain seems overwhelming, but it will pass if you are willing to identify and own it. Feelings are transitory; they pass. As intense as your pain can be, trying to control and defend against your feelings prolongs the pain. Allow yourself to own them and be with them.

The following are some suggestions to begin this process of owning your feelings.

- **Journal.** Carry a notebook with you. Throughout the day or at a specific time every day, write about what you've been feeling.

- **Create a feelings list.** Make a list of feelings and carry it with you. Bring it out three times daily and ask yourself what you have been feeling. For example: "I am feeling guilty about I am feeling sad about _____." "I am feeling afraid about _____." "I am feeling angry about _____." "I am feeling embarrassed about _____." Share what you are feeling with someone you trust.

- **Affirm your emotional self.** Identify two affirmations that will support you in acknowledging your feelings. For example: "I have the right to my feelings" and "My feelings help me identify my needs."

- **Breathe deeply.** People close off their feelings when they take shallow breaths. Check your breathing throughout the day and particularly at times of vulnerability. Take a deep breath in for three seconds, exhale slowly for three seconds; repeat five times. In time expand this to five seconds, five times.

Recognizing Yourself in the Grief Process

A lot of what you are experiencing is the accumulation of many years of unacknowledged feelings related to loss and grief. Think about the losses you suffered because of your partner's sexual acting out. Some losses may include:

- He wasn't there for the birth of a child.

- He acted out the night before your wedding.

- He had a child with another woman and he didn't tell you for years.

- He hid money from you.

- He spent money on other women.

- He didn't show up to a lot of family activities.

- He told lies, lies, and more lies.

- He blamed you for not being sexual enough.

- He was not present when he was with you; his thoughts were focused elsewhere.

The classic grief model encompasses a series of universal emotional reactions. The model always starts with loss, but from there it is not necessarily linear. It encompasses shock. You are numb to what occurred; you disbelieve. Denial is only human. When your loss is too painful to acknowledge you move into denial. You minimize, rationalize. In order to get to acceptance, you move through anger. And you have so much to be angry about. Somewhere in the process guilt sets in and that leads to bargaining. This bargaining is often between you and your God or Higher Power: "God, if you would just make him stop this behavior, I promise I will_____." Then you experience sorrow, the sadness deep and profound. You feel too helpless to respond. With progress through these stages, you come to acceptance, acceptance of the reality for what it is.

When loss is chronic and the likelihood of abandonment looms at emotionally painful times, you are more apt to bypass the shock stage of grief and quickly proceed to the denial stage. If you have made a habit of employing denial to cope with your feelings, you have become so skilled at this that you may have difficulty even identifying a situation as a loss. You may think the following:

- *No, it wasn't important to me that my husband didn't get to my awards banquet last night. I really didn't expect him to show up.*

- *I am used to it. It didn't really hurt.*

- *I suspected he was out at the strip club, but I told myself as long as he was with his work buddies it was okay.*

Anger is a natural response to loss. It is a protest, an attempt to retrieve what is gone or never was. Feeling anger can be a healthy reaction when your rights have been stomped on. It heightens your awareness and propels you to act. Without it you may lack the courage to speak out, to seek a just resolution, and to protect yourself from further harm. If you don't allow yourself to feel indignant when someone hurts you, if you don't know that you are bruised or enraged, who will encourage you to question what your relationship is worth? Who will draw the line and say enough is enough? Who will be your voice? Inability to feel anger is as dangerous as the inability to feel pain and it will render you just as defenseless. Acknowledging pain allows you to address it. When you have been hurt, anger is a natural, valid response. It can be a gift, as it provides a feeling of empowerment. Suddenly you do not doubt yourself. You can do whatever needs to be done. Anger gives you energy to cope; it reinforces your confidence and offers the strength to mobilize. Anger's vector is always forward—to push away the source of pain. In anger it is easier to forget the other person's needs. All that counts is your pain and your needs, not theirs. The partner who has been more in tune to other people's needs than her own can be mobilized by anger to act on her own behalf.

But when you are afraid of rejection, distrust your own perceptions, and are highly dependent on others' approval, you have difficulty owning your anger. You don't want to be angry; you want to be understanding. That's anger avoidance. When you are anger avoidant you find it easier to skip the anger stage of grieving and move straight on to guilt or depression. Inability to identify anger interferes with your ability to move through the grief process.

If you are chronically angry, on the other hand, you may be stuck in the grief process, unable to move from your anger. Anger is your safe place; other feelings are the ones that create greater vulnerability for you. A very important question then is: What would you be feeling if you weren't angry?

Guilt (both true and false) is a natural response to a loss. *True guilt* is a feeling of regret or remorse over something you have or have not done. *False guilt* is the feeling of regret or remorse for someone else's behavior and actions. If you have difficulty separating true guilt from false guilt, you are more apt to stay stuck. As a result, you continue to wonder what you could have done to have made things different: "If I had paid more attention to him . . ." or "If I did what he wanted sexually . . ." or "If I had been home more . . ." The false guilt you carry keeps you stuck in the bargaining stage. As painful as it is for anyone to wend his or her way through a grief process, many people find a type of psychological safety in their bargaining. To let go of the bargaining and reach a healthy place of acceptance, you have to allow yourself to acknowledge and tolerate very intense feelings. If this is difficult for you, don't despair. In recovery you will develop the ability to tolerate your feelings without engaging in self-defeating or otherwise self-destructive behavior.

Sorrow is a normal part of the grief process. There is so much to feel sorrow about. It can feel overwhelming. When you think that you aren't worthy, you are apt to succumb to the power of defeat and experience a more chronic state of depression rather than move on to acceptance.

When you are grieving, it is not the time to be judgmental or critical about what it is you are feeling. You've been wounded and you're hurt; your feelings are legitimate.

Acceptance comes as a result of having been able to experience each step of the grief process. Acceptance does not mean what your partner has done is okay or not hurtful. It means accepting the reality of his behavior and its impact on you, your relationship, and your family. Finding meaning for yourself from this experience is significant in your healing process.

Review the dynamics of loss and grief—shock, denial, anger, guilt, bargaining, sorrow, and acceptance—and identify where you are more apt to get mired in the process. While shock and denial are often the first stages of grief, you will find that you will slip in and out of the other feelings, frequently revisiting them. Depending on your defenses, you are also more likely to stay in some stages longer than others.

Getting through the grief process takes time, but people who actively engage in their recovery find that the pain gradually diminishes. In times of intense feelings, you need to take deliberate steps to lessen your external stresses. Be aware that you are in a vulnerable emotional state, and it is going to be important for you to identify and practice self-care behaviors. That means you need to eat healthy, get some exercise, rest properly, and take advantage of a support system. This is no time to take on added responsibilities. Make more time for yourself. Stay aware that you are vulnerable. There is no specific time frame allotted to complete your grief process. Don't put expectations or shoulds on yourself. With the help of others in recovery and/or a professional, you'll find you're able to work through your grief in your own time. It is a passage that does not last forever. Now is the time to treat yourself gently and with kindness.

How Long Will It Hurt?

I liken the process of grieving over losses to peeling an onion. You do it one layer at a time, and in the process you cry a lot.

You may cry until your eyes swell shut and your bones ache. One day you think you are doing okay and the next day you feel devastation again. The losses are so deep: the ability to trust, your dreams, your confidence, the sanctity of your marriage bed, the blow to your pride. The pain often comes in waves. At times numbness may move in and out. This is very common as the truth unfolds. Numbness is protective and temporary. You will be able to experience a wider range and greater depth of feelings, as you begin to feel increasingly safer.

[PARTNER]

The pain comes and goes as I'm in recovery. It's true the pain is not like it was in the beginning, and I often feel as if I'm moving to different levels of pain.

Sometimes I feel overwhelmed because so much of my life I've stayed away from anger and sadness. I used to just put my feelings in a drawer and move to a happier me. I know it was a mask, but learning how to swim in anger and sadness makes me vulnerable and I don't like it. My recovery support and practices help me embrace the pain and take care of myself.

Your pain is both deep and wide. Sadly, we haven't invented a healthy remedy to make it go away quickly. Quick fixes only lead to a deeper, longer fracture later. While feelings don't disappear, the intensity of them will decrease if you give voice to all of them. They also lessen when your partner does his part and works on repairing the damage. Whether or not he joins you in the recovery process, your pain will lessen when you accept the reality of what has happened. It lessens, as you own your pain, your shame, and your anger. You need to live with the pain, accept its reality, and practice healthy behavior until the hurt begins to ease.

It may be helpful to think of grief as a hurricane-force wind. If you stand rigid, lock your knees, support your back with a broom, and keep your feet together, the wind will surely blow you over. Conversely, if you stand and face the wind with balance and flexibility, with space between your feet, knees bent, and leaning into the wind, you may sway like a palm tree on the beach, but you will find your strength and durability. Peace comes by walking through the pain, not around it. The process of grieving and attending to your losses will take months, and you will periodically find yourself back in the grief process when a specific issue is triggered—even years into your recovery journey. The depth and span of your suffering is strongly influenced by the degree of grief you allow yourself to experience in early recovery.

It is crucial that you have a support system, people you can talk with regularly about these feelings. Talking, rather than keeping the feelings inside, takes the power out of the feelings. It is essential for you to find other people who understand your circumstances and to listen to their stories, too. Eventually you will be better able to share your story. Receiving validation from others lessens your pain.

Your Sexual Relationship

While some couples insist their sexual relationship has been strong aside from the addiction, when both partners are in recovery, the emotional and relational tools they learned will enhance and change the previous experiences to one of greater intimacy. As Chapter Five described, a celibacy contract is strongly advised in early recovery and before a sexual relationship is resumed.

[ADDICT]

Our initial sexual relationship started with me bringing her into my addictions, so in recovery our sex life had to start all over. I had to learn the basics of holding hands; then we had dates where we did fun things together. We went to ball games. We hiked. During those times we held hands, we kissed on the lips, small kisses. We touched knees. We talked about little things and big things. Then we talked about how we felt after the date. Some of this sounds silly but it was great.

The steps the addict above described allowed this couple to develop a friendship; it inspired a sense of loving romance into their marriage. It created safe environments to be together and talk with each other. It allowed both partners and the coupleship to grow intimately.

Like many women who have been socialized to feel sexually shy, the woman who shares below is learning to honor her needs rather than predominantly focus on her partner's needs.

[PARTNER]

I always accepted what he said was good sex, what he liked. So while I had the physical part down, I needed to learn to tell him what I liked. I had to take risks by speaking up and taking ownership of what made me feel good versus focusing on his needs. He had to deal with his insecurity about thinking he was supposed to know what pleasured me and that somehow there was something wrong if I redirected him. We read books together about healthy sexuality and I think because we both really wanted to have this part of our relationship better, we stayed with it and today it is much better.

In the recovery process this partner learns to take more ownership of her sexual desires and needs, and the addict has the opportunity to share rather than to control the experience, creating intimacy.

In the past, addiction overshadowed any healthy sexual experiences, and you were likely responding to the socialization of who you are and how you are supposed to act sexually. The addict did not have healthy sexual esteem in his active addiction, and it doesn't suddenly exist just because he has quit acting out. Now, in recovery, you both bring a vulnerability to this intimate experience. You are still experiencing the feelings of a relationship that has been seriously hurt.

[PARTNER]

My husband acts scared of being sexual with me. I can feel his tentativeness, his anxiety, and then I get anxious and frustrated. Then we get in this pattern of not even trying to be sexual.

This is a critical time when unspoken thoughts and feelings sabotage the reconnection. Keep communicating.

At any point in the recovery process where sex is being avoided, it is time to again consider an agreement for a therapeutic sexual time out. During this time you're working as a couple to identify and address the barriers and resistances to sexual intimacy.

It is possible that one or both of you may experience a phenomenon of the addictive cycle called *sexual anorexia*. Sexual anorexia is a dread or self-hate of one's sexuality. Yet the term is used broadly and may also be defined as a fear of intimacy to the point where the person has severe anxiety surrounding sex.

[ADDICT]

In my addiction I was nonsexual with my girlfriend but completely out of control with one-night affairs, prostitutes, phone sex, massage parlors, and the internet.

I am in recovery today, meaning I don't do those things anymore but I still avoid my partner sexually. It is not about her. Maybe her not pushing me to be sexual is about her, but I hate what I have done, that whole part of me, and when I try to be sexual with her I am impotent or I ejaculate prematurely. I am like a scared young boy. Not exactly the vision of a sex addict, is it? Ever since I was a child I have felt that I am bad for feeling sexual and should be punished.

Switching to polar opposite behaviors often reflects the extremes of living with addiction. As the addict may experience sexual anorexia, you may fluctuate in your behavior, being flagrantly sexual in an attempt to combat your severe dislike of your sexual self to blatantly avoiding sexual behaviors. This is similar to the binge-purge cycle of a bulimic where he or she overeats and then purges the food. It is also possible to simply move to one side of the continuum and stay there in a more purely anorexic, deprived state. Regardless of the pattern, binge or purge, recovery involves learning and valuing healthy sexuality and addressing the loss and trauma issues that underlie this severe reaction to one's sexuality.

[PARTNER]

As much as I hated knowing he was sexual with others, in some ways I was relieved to not be sexual. I had never liked that part of me. For years I wouldn't confront him about what I knew he was doing because then he wouldn't ask much from me.

To help you understand the framework, the following are indicators of healthy sexuality:

- Accepts the imperfect.

- Adds to self-esteem.

- Has no victims.

- Holds integrity.

- Is fun and playful.

- Is mutual.

- Maintains respect.

- Relies on safety.

Undoubtedly, the key to healthy sexuality for you and the addict begins with emotional healing. When there is so much anger, shame, and pain, you need to be realistic and patient in your expectations. Conversations about what is satisfying and emotionally safe for both partners need to occur and keep occurring throughout your coupleship. As you build your adult-to-adult relationship around spiritually and emotionally healthy guidelines, the physical aspect of your relationship can become a more enriching experience.

Facing Relapse

What if he acts out again? Reengaging in the behavior after some recovery practice is referred to as *relapse*. Unfortunately the possibility is always there, and relapses occur for many in the recovery process. In a treatment process or a twelve-step program, the addict will have defined for himself what sexual sobriety entails and that will vary depending on how he acted out. It could mean he will not use the internet to access sexual sites or it could mean he'll not use the internet at all. He might decide that he can still masturbate or that masturbation is not allowed. He will have identified what is a part of his addiction cycle, and he will be accountable for what triggers him to act out.

Most women find that with some time in recovery, they look at any relapse in its overall context. What was the behavior? How did the addict respond to having a relapse? How quickly did he tell you and others to whom he is accountable about the relapse? In what ways was he accountable? What is he doing to prevent a future relapse? Is he asking himself what he needs to do or address in his recovery that he was not attending to or previously addressing enough?

One woman became aware her partner was watching sexual videos and masturbating. He told both his twelve-step sponsor (a chosen mentor in his twelve-step program) and her within a couple of days of his relapse. In her mind he was being accountable by quickly owning his behavior and having some insight into what triggered it. He also had a plan to handle the trigger differently should it occur again. She expressed her disappointment, fear, and anger about his behavior, but realized it was his to address and that she would stay focused on her recovery.

Therese was confronted with her husband's relapsing when he began using pornography again and then sought out women at a massage parlor. He had been relapsing about every four months, which involved pornography on the internet, but this behavior was a major escalation from that. By then he had been in recovery for a few years and his relapses were like binge drinking—periods of being dry and then a short period of acting out on a cyclical basis. This relapse led to a therapeutic separation for the couple. The consequence here appears more severe, but in the overall context, they both saw this relapse as a threat to his long-term recovery and their marriage, and they felt a therapeutic separation would help them better address their individual recovery issues.

You have choices about how you respond to known relapses. How you think you will respond and how you actually respond may vary. That is most likely dependent on your history with the addict and how much more you are willing to tolerate. You may feel there is no room for any relapse or the relationship will end, and that is your bottom line. Women whom I have worked with had the greatest difficulty with relapses when the relapse included physical contact with another or that had legal ramifications. Relapses that include masturbation, viewing porn, or attending a strip joint may be more forgivable. But all relapses are serious because they create distortion in your relationship; they set up a disconnection between the two of you and may trigger escalating behavior on his part. It may offer some comfort to believe you know exactly how you'd handle a relapse should it occur. However, I suggest you not try to problem-solve and don't live in the future of "what ifs." If you are in your own healing process, you will have the tools to address a relapse should it occur.

As the addict may experience relapse, partners do as well. You will find it helpful in your healing to recognize the reengagement of self-defeating thoughts and behaviors as your own relapse. Your relapse means returning to a pattern of behavior, such as resuming your detective behavior, saying yes to situations when you really want to say no, or verbal raging.

What would your relapse behaviors be?

Remember that recovery is a process; you are learning new ways of thinking and relating. This process takes time, so you don't need to be harsh on yourself.

Building Trust

Your partner can verbalize his intentions for fidelity; he can be honest in the moment. But the only guarantee is that there are no guarantees. This issue confronts every partner who is new to recovery. Of course you'd like reassurance; you want to be able to trust that you're getting the truth, but this will take time. Women become more trusting of their partners when they see them engage in recovery practices, when they see a commitment to continuing therapy or participation in self-help groups. Trust comes when that commitment to recovery practice translates into changes in behavior, such as fewer angry outbursts, less controlling behavior, consistency in behavior, dependability, and accountability. It comes when he is open to answering questions, not resentful of engaging recovery practices; when he demonstrates an ability to empathize with your feelings, especially about his past behaviors. Time plus change in behavior will be the building blocks to developing trust in your relationship.

[THERESE]

Time, sobriety, and working the program will help me to have more trust. I don't expect to ever trust completely again. But I can live with that. It isn't as tough as it sounds; maybe I just have less illusion about the human condition.

The fact that Therese says she can live with no absolutes of trust is only possible because of her recovery. She can live with no guarantees because she is accepting of the gifts of recovery. For so many women, life in early recovery means living in limbo and ambiguity. It is hard to keep moving forward when the future of your coupleship is not totally within your power. But it never is and never was. The illusion may feel secure, but again, it's an illusion. Recovery will lead you to restoring or developing your self-esteem, improving communication, and trusting yourself to do what is right for you. It is in your recovery process that you will choose to be accountable for your own health, practicing relational skills of knowing and speaking your feelings, thoughts, and needs. You speak to be accountable for yourself; you listen to better know your partner. You learn to set healthy boundaries wherein you do not forsake your own esteem. You learn to trust in your own perceptions, your own internal voice—a voice you discounted or minimized for years.

[MAITE]

It doesn't matter if I trust him, I trust myself. If I have a feeling, an intuition, or something doesn't feel right, today I make sure I say it. Before, it was about not trusting me, not just him. I would be too quiet. It's not okay now not to be heard. He is on his journey and I see him going to his therapy and his meetings, doing his exercise, and that is helping to assure me that he takes care of himself.

[JACQUE]

In early recovery I had this great need to know. I thought if I was up on everything that was going on in his mind, heard about every thought in his addictive thinking, and knew about how he dealt with every temptation, then I would be able to control the situation. Later I learned that this is a part of my own illness. Today I look at his commitment to his twelve-step program, attendance at meetings, and a change in attitude as signs of recovery. I have found I may come to trust certain things 100 percent, but other things will not be so clear.

[JENNY]

I am not in control of what will happen, and I
learn to give my fears to God.

These women are practicing the act of "letting go." Letting go
is a spiritual concept.

André Gide wrote, "One does not discover new lands without
consenting to lose sight of the shore for a very long time."[2] Letting
go, relinquishing the need for control, the need to be right, and
the need to be all-knowing means you genuinely accept in your
heart that holding on to old behavior holds no promise; it does not
work and it does not help. For many, a willingness to be in this in-
between state only becomes doable with the alliance of a spiritual
path. Chapter Eight will give you the opportunity to reflect on
how spiritual practice can be significant to your healing.

Asking for Help

You probably have been coping on your own or with the advice
and direction of family and friends. Hopefully the time has come
for you to let go of your fears and shame and be willing to get help
from a professional or recovery program that specifically addresses
your issues. You don't need to wait for your partner to be willing
to get help; you don't even need to be in the relationship any longer
for you to get help. Regardless of the status of the relationship
you are left with, the trauma of the betrayal, depression, anxiety,
and a host of self-defeating behaviors could be governing your life.
Your foundational beliefs about your self-worth and value are in
question. Perhaps your own addictions have come to light. Signs of
post-traumatic stress may become apparent, as well as the role of
childhood wounding and trauma repetition.

You deserve the opportunity to work with someone, privately
or in a group, who can lead and support you. Professional and self-
help resources are out there. Look for a therapist who has specific
training in how to work with family members families impacted by

sex addiction. You are most apt to find them via the International Institute for Trauma and Addiction Professionals (IITAP) affiliated with the Society for the Advancement of Sexual Health (SASH), or the Association of Partners of Sex Addicts Trauma Specialist (APSATS). Talk with others who have struggled with the same problems and who have sought the help of a professional. Find out what they valued or did not value about their choice of therapist before you call for an appointment. Also if it is difficult to find someone locally it is much more common today to work with someone via the internet, with Skype and/or other media platforms.

While I have a strong bias for the opportunity for partners to work with other partners in a group, it could be difficult to find a group in your community. If that is the case, I strongly encourage you, if feasible, to locate a partners workshop that would give you at least a one time experience with other partners. This is most often a three- to five-day group experience. It is always best if you are already working with a therapist individually who works with you prior and after a workshop experience. See Helping Resources for suggestions.

Because of the traumatic stress that is experienced it is most helpful to also find a therapist that incorporates trauma modalities into his or her practice. Such modalities that many partners have found helpful range from Somatic Experiencing (SE), Eye Movement Desensitization Reprocessing (EMDR), forms of mindfulness practice, art therapies, sensorimotor psychotherapy (SP), and others. It is common that many therapists associated with the above clinical techniques have such training or are familiar with clinicians to whom they could refer you. You don't have to be familiar with these modalities as much as to not be surprised and to be open to them when suggested.

Be open to exploring specific twelve-step programs for partners of sex addicts. S-Anon and COSA groups are more prevalent than the lesser known Codependents of Sex and Love Addicts Anonymous (COSLAA). The focus of these groups is specific to partners of sex addicts. Recovering Couples Anonymous (RCA) is also a viable twelve-step program for couples to attend together.

Because these meetings are held primarily in larger urban areas, and thus unavailable to some, many women will need to find a program of recovery in the programs of Al-Anon, Codependents Anonymous, and Adult Children of Alcoholics. Al-Anon offers a strong basis for "staying on your side of the sidewalk"—taking responsibility for yourself without being preoccupied with your partner's behavior. The latter two groups will help you focus directly on codependency and family of origin issues. Twelve-step meetings are peer led with no professional facilitation and no fees. Confidentiality and anonymity are strongly enforced. They are structured on the traditions and recovery steps of the original successful model of Alcoholics Anonymous.

See Helpful Resources to find a list of websites that will be helpful in seeking professional and/or self-help services.

[JACQUE]

In the beginning I drove two hundred miles round-trip to find a self-help group for partners of sex addicts. After several months in both this group and in Al-Anon in my hometown, I started one group in my own community. I practically ran to a group looking for hope and help with how to live with this problem. I was looking for connections with others who would validate my feelings, women whose lives looked like mine.

Reflect back on the women who introduced themselves in Chapter One. In their journeys all of them found a place in a group. Some of them entered a specific therapy group for spouses and/or partners of sex addicts; others connected in a twelve-step group. Initially the only thing they knew about these groups was that there would be other women and possibly men there who had spouses and/or partners who identified as sex addicts.

[THERESE]

I couldn't believe that I was so desperate that I would take myself to this group of people who supposedly had the same type of problems I was having. How could that be? When I felt my whole family disintegrating, with pressure from my counselor I was willing to do anything that might take away my horrendous pain. To think that life is full of so many hidden secrets. And then I began to hear others and realized they were the mirror image of me. My pain was at least temporarily set aside as I felt both shock and relief to know I was not alone.

[VANESSA]

I was so scared, confused, and uncertain of my marriage. I was intimidated by the words "sex addiction." How strange to be intimidated. After all, sex addiction was what I was living with. I found myself driving around in any and all directions, not sure why I was going in the direction I was. I finally had the sense to pull the car over, stop, and try to figure out what I was doing. Odd, but in essence, it's what I needed to do with my life.

[SARA]

I walked into the group room full of anger and fury about what my husband was doing. I was in absolute terror about my future and the future of my family, both financially and emotionally. The fear was overwhelming.

I was in horrible pain about the choices and mistakes I had made, the shame about our situation. I knew I didn't know all of the facts. I would go through more shocks, hurt, shame, and outrage. And it was in that room that I would find a way out of my shame and pain.

[JENNY]

Here I was walking into this group of women who had partners or husbands like mine. Men who flagrantly, yet deceivingly, had been with other women in lots of different ways—women in massage parlors, women at work, even women who were supposedly friends. I had been living in a capsule for so long, drifting at sea, being tossed around in a storm. I was ready to no longer be alone.

I cannot emphasize enough the healing power of a group—whether it is a self-help group or therapy group—of women who have experiences similar to yours. In both twelve-step groups and therapy, confidentiality is strongly adhered to. I know you probably feel ashamed and angry and don't want to be exposed. You think this is a private issue and may be concerned about your family's anonymity. Yet it is in the group experience that many women heal to a degree they never imagined possible. In the group they come to realize their healing journey is a gift to themselves that will take them through life and its ultimate challenges.

Even though you have read how many women found answers in a group setting you may still find yourself procrastinating. "Yes, but . . ." "Yes, but I have childcare problems." "Yes, but I have transportation problems." Or "Yes, but I am very well known and visible in my community and couldn't possibly expose myself like that."

Stop. Take a deep breath. Prioritize your well-being, as it affects every aspect of your life. I know you don't want to keep living with stress and shame. Perhaps your unwillingness to reach out to others is because you don't want to intrude; maybe you think you've imposed enough on those people closest to you. Your fear of being burdensome is an aspect of your codependency and is detrimental to your welfare. You deserve better; you deserve more. If childcare is a concern, think about asking a family member or trusted friend to sit with your children. If transportation is your problem, seek out community resources or public transportation. A twelve-step member will often offer to help you get to a meeting. If you maintain a high profile in your community and you feel that the visibility of participating in a group would greatly impact other areas of your life, know that the anonymity at twelve-step meetings is sacred, and confidentiality is required in therapy with a professional. Also, here in the United States there are specialists in the sex addiction field working with many high-profile individuals and couples. But it is mostly fear and shame that will keep you away. As you allow your reality to be acknowledged, the fear and shame will lessen.

Your time to heal has come. It won't happen all at once; it will be a process. There will continue to be obstacles to overcome, pain to face, and work to do. Yet on your journey of healing, you'll gain the strength to walk through the pain. You'll learn to own your voice, identify your feelings, and grieve your losses. You will come to terms with your powerlessness over your partner's addictive behavior and recognize where your personal power lies. It lies with your own behavior and your choices. The work you'll do—establishing boundaries and letting go of the need to control—will be a freeing experience that increases your sense of who you are and what you need and want. This will give you the courage to be the person you want to be, who you truly are. You will feel your value and worth and come to embrace the need for self-care, knowing it is an act of self-love. You deserve that. And you don't need to do this alone. Addiction and living in the betrayal zone are about isolation, disconnection from self and others. Recovery is about connection. Allow others to be a part of this journey.

Reflective Thoughts and Questions

- Do you agree that it is your time to heal? What does that mean to you?

- What boundaries would help you at this time in your recovery?

- What can you do to lessen your rumination?

- Which feelings do you have difficulty expressing?

- How would you describe yourself in the grief process?

- What self-defeating thoughts and behaviors would you identify as relapse indicators for you?

- Where does your power lie?

- Have you been willing to ask for help? Do you need more assistance?

- What was important for you to learn in this chapter?

CHAPTER SEVEN NOTES

1   The Serenity Prayer was written by Reinhold Niebuhr (1892–1971): "God, grant me the serenity to accept the things I cannot change, the courage to change the things I can, and the wisdom to know the difference."

2   André Gide. French critic, essayist, and novelist (1869–1951). Source of quote unknown.

CHAPTER EIGHT

Finding Your Serenity

Can I ever forgive him?

How do I find peace?

With every tear you shed and every outcry of rage you release, more room is opened in your heart for forgiveness and a sense of peace to enter. As you progress in your own journey of recovery, you will likely contemplate forgiveness and what that means for you. You will develop a deeper connection with God or a Higher Power. And you will discover your own spiritual path. These are all ways to support your healing process.

Forgiveness

Women have been taught that they owe it to others to forgive their transgressions. But there are no "shoulds" here. The addict often asks for your forgiveness soon after you've heard the news. Frequently women who immediately offer forgiveness to their partners are engaging in what we refer to as *cheap* or *false forgiveness*—an act that deepens the denial process by promoting an illusion of closeness when nothing has changed, has been faced, or has been resolved. You may want to dismiss the injury to yourself and the relationship for the sake of protecting it. Your record and habit of being overly compliant and going to great lengths to avoid conflict is entrenched. In her book *How Can I Forgive You?* Janis Spring eloquently describes cheap forgiveness as trying to preserve a relationship at any cost, including sacrificing your integrity and safety. On the surface you may act as if nothing is wrong, but inside you're bleeding out. Silencing your anguish and indignation only silences your heart and soul.[1]

FALSE FORGIVENESS

To avoid disrupting the relationship with expectations or boundaries, cheap forgiveness may come readily to you. Perhaps a deep fear of conflict and anger, the fear of rejection and abandonment, or the strong need for outside approval fuel your desire to quickly forgive. With a smile on your face, you remain in the relationship without a voice and with minimal expectations. Or you leave the relationship only to reengage in another, repeating your pattern. Once again, you don't ask, you don't expect, and you don't operate from a place of esteem or worth, but from a place of defeat or silent defiance.

[THERESE]

I was so busy doing what I thought was right. I thought I forgave my husband. I said the words; I smiled. Well, there is no right here. Of course I knew I was hurt. I was angry, but I was working so hard to not be angry. I thought that made me look bad and I wanted him to be the bad person; after all, his behavior was the problem. I just couldn't tolerate being out of control with my feelings, which is how I feel when I'm angry. So I smiled and talked forgiveness and then silently punished him as much as I could. I was still living inside his addiction.

[MAITE]

Before recovery I did a lot of false forgiveness. I pretended to forgive, but I kept a secret file with all the information about his lovers and acting-out behaviors just in case, and I would gossip about his behavior with others.

[JENNY]

Prior to my beginning any specific recovery, I had a lot of years of false forgiveness. Mostly it was just going numb and trying to breathe. But after recovery began and I really understood what we were both dealing with, he would badger me by telling me I had to forgive him because, after all, he was changing. But it was badgering, and it was not a lot different from his old behavior. A bit softer in volume, but the tone was still a threat to me. Somehow it was like if I would say the words, "I forgive you," then I didn't have the right to have any limits or ask for things to be different.

You won't get to a place of heartfelt forgiveness without being emotionally honest. When you say you forgive but you have not claimed your voice, not grieved your pain, and not owned the injustice, then you're only talking the talk but not walking the walk of recovery.

I worked briefly with a woman who was not willing to stay in the therapy process or to ask her husband to look seriously at his behavior. They had been married for twenty-five years, and during all those years he blatantly acted out with other women, flaunting them in her face. She spent all those years in the act of cheap forgiveness. She didn't believe her husband's repetitive sexual acting out was addictive, but even more she didn't think he had any responsibility for his behavior. She frequently caught him in his lies and deceit, and she forgave him time after time after time. She thought, *He really does love me; it's just those other women.* Her vision focused only on his woman of the moment. She was convinced that as long as the other women stayed away, she and her husband were just fine. He did love her; it was just that those other women came in as if from outer space and captured him against his will.

FORGIVENESS AND RECOVERY

Being able or willing to forgive is not the focus of recovery. If you have just become aware of the nature of your partner's behavior, you are still grieving significant losses. Forgiveness at this point would be very premature and most likely false—again, cheap forgiveness. The process of true forgiveness begins with acknowledging that a wrong has been done to you. Then you can grieve; you can own the feelings associated with those wrongs, and that certainly means owning your anger and pain. You pursue your own recovery, set boundaries, and decide which behaviors in the relationship you can and cannot accept.

Whether or not the relationship is sustained, the act of forgiving is about your own healing; it is about letting go of resentments, preoccupation, and controlling behavior. Far too often when there is a separation or divorce the partner holds on to her resentments. I've met many women who, years later, are still consumed with resentments pertaining to their previous partner. This negativity in their life that comes with obsessive resentment darkens every other relationship, be it with their children, friends, coworkers, or new partners.

Forgiveness is a moral right, not your moral obligation. Love does not obligate you. Ultimately, forgiveness is remembering and letting go. It is about being true to you. So don't put a timetable on this. Don't put any "shoulds" onto yourself. Forgiveness is made possible with your commitment to your own recovery practices.

It may offer you some peace of mind while you are in this journey to have a framework for forgiveness. Only in knowing what that means can you put it into a healing perspective. Think about the following aspects of forgiveness.

When you forgive, you no longer build an identity around something that happened to you. You realize that there is more to you than your history with your partner. The past is put into its proper perspective as one part of who you are in the present.

When you forgive, you recognize that you no longer need your grudges and resentments, your hatred, your self-pity. You don't need these negative emotions as excuses for getting less out of life than you want or deserve. You do not need them as a weapon to hurt those who hurt you or to keep other people from getting close enough to hurt you again. You no longer want to punish the people who hurt you. You realize that you truly do not want to even the score; forgiveness is the inner peace you feel when you stop trying to do so.

[PARTNER]

I found my way to forgiveness when I began to set boundaries and tell my boyfriend what I needed from him. I asked for very specific things, and when he responded positively it softened my heart. I asked him to talk to the children, who were seventeen and twenty. I knew they knew a lot, but technically it was still all a big secret. I was looking like the bad guy because I was so angry and depressed. So together we sat and talked to them. We did that with some guidelines from a counselor. It took a lot of courage and I am grateful. I asked that he change departments at work and he did that. He didn't want to but he did it anyway. I was just too upset all of the time to know he was working next to one of the people he acted out with. I asked him to change his cell phone number. I asked a lot of things and he actually did them. That was all part of the process, but I think his willingness to hear me and to respect my requests helped make it possible for me to begin to forgive.

[SARA]

Forgiveness is the most challenging thing of all. Well, forgiveness and trust. I have learned over the years that forgiveness is a process totally about me, not about another person. It's about what I want for myself. In the Big Book of Alcoholics Anonymous it is suggested that what you want for yourself, you pray for your enemy. I believe that forgiveness is manifested through prayer for his or her well-being. That is how I have come to forgiveness.

[MAITE]

Real forgiveness started for me when, through education and being in therapy groups with addicts and their partners, I was able to see this as a compulsive disorder that affected his brain and hijacked his will and his soul and, in that process, mine, too. It is not about me or even him. As I call it, it is a cancer of the soul, our souls. We are a wounded couple, thirsty for healing. That was the beginning of compassion, true compassion, and a lot of grieving for me, for him, for our families, our losses, our lives. It was not about judging; it was about getting control of a disorder that was destroying us, not only during crisis, but on a daily basis. Soon after that I started having glimpses of the gifts of the pain and that was the beginning of my new spirituality.

[VANESSA]

Coming from a highly religious background, I think I had a warped viewpoint of forgiveness; high levels of judgment were a part of the formula followed by mandated forgiveness, which simply meant bury it. Operating from this misguided viewpoint of forgiveness just made me more toxic. I would forgive him verbally and then throw it back in his face at the first sign of trouble. It fed my superiority and confusion. It also kept me in a dangerous place of denying the resentment. You can't heal from what you don't own. I first had to experience the pain rather than medicate it through busyness or helping others. As a perpetual happy-face wife, I had to get to the root of my anger and do some releasing. "It was hard work, considering it was buried so deep. But a wonderful freedom comes from congruence and authenticity! Upon experiencing and feeling honest emotions, I was then able to release it.

A very valuable tool for me to come to a place of genuine forgiveness with both my husband's acting out and my father's raging behavior was to start seeing them in their own woundedness; realizing they were not participating in these behaviors to be mean to me, but because they were broken. Hurt people hurt people. In one of my groups, we were led through a visualization in which we got in touch with our inner child. Then we were to see our abuser as a child as well. In the exercise we introduced the two pure little children and I visualized them walking off together hand in hand, unfettered by the pains that drove their adult actions. It was a beautiful way for me to see them for who they were at their core rather than simply by their actions. This was another step to letting go of the resentments and anger I was carrying and to honor the soul instead of continuing to focus on the behavior. To this day I find this exercise very helpful when I can't seem to get past a behavior that disturbs me.

It may be easier to appreciate what forgiveness is by recognizing what forgiveness is not. The following thoughts may be helpful to you as you sort through your feelings and come to terms with the role of forgiveness in your healing.

Forgiveness is not forgetting what has happened. Your past experiences and pain have a great deal to teach you about not being victimized again and about not victimizing others. Forgiving the people who hurt you does not mean you condone or absolve them of their behavior. You are not saying that what was done to you was acceptable or unimportant or was not hurtful. It was important, it hurt, and it has made a difference in your life. Forgiveness doesn't erase what he has done. He is still responsible for the harm his behavior has created.

Forgiveness doesn't mean you are never angry again about what occurred. What happened to you was not right; it was not fair. For that you may always feel anger. You have every reason and right to be angry. But you want to get to a point where your anger no longer interferes with how you care about yourself or how you live your life.

Forgiveness doesn't happen by making a one-time decision. No matter how sincerely you want to let go of the past and move on with your life, you cannot just wave a magic wand or flip a switch and blithely make the past disappear in one moment.

[JACQUE]

What he did was not okay. I hated him for it. I trusted him because I wanted so badly for him to be my knight in shining armor. Now I know I blindly trusted. It's been a couple of years now in recovery for both of us, and I have forgiven him. My ability to forgive him came as I found my strength. I set boundaries I had never previously had. I owned feelings I have spent my life avoiding. As I started to take care of me and think about me, I insisted on recovery practices for the marriage that I hoped would ensure our relationship. As he moved forward in recovery, I could be more compassionate to who he was. But during this time I did not focus on wanting to forgive him. That wasn't even in my realm of thinking. I was just trying to make sense out of what had happened in my life. I didn't want to live with self-loathing and pain. I came to understand us in a way I hadn't before. We are lucky as we were both in search of wholeness, which ultimately has only been found in our recovery. From that strength of being more whole, I could come to the place of forgiveness.

Forgiveness doesn't mean reconciliation. Sometimes you fight against any form of forgiveness because you think that means you have to stay in the relationship. Reconciliation is a choice. You may choose to leave the relationship, or he may opt out. Whether or not the relationship survives, the recovery process is your opportunity to let go of self-defeating thoughts, feelings, and behaviors; to learn new relational skills; and garner esteem from within. Too often the relationship ends, and even if that is your choice, you stay angry and depressed and continue to act in ways that erode your esteem. That does not have to be you.

[JENNY]

After some time in recovery there was this quiet acceptance. I didn't know if I forgave him, but I quit hating him. I started to see him differently. He was no longer this monster to me. Yet I chose to divorce after a couple of years of us working a recovery program. Not letting him back into my life in a committed relationship had nothing to do with forgiving or not forgiving him, it had to do with boundaries. I found we had too little foundation and I could feel no love. I can get philosophical at times about what our journey together was about. I go in and out of times when I feel anger about the years we spent together, being hurtful toward ourselves and each other. I still have to deal with him around our kids, and I find myself judgmental and critical—I am not perfect by any means. I realize I am human. How is that for self-forgiveness? Today I am more at peace than ever, not because I am not with him anymore but because I chose to quit hanging on to my resentments and my wounds. What freedom it gave me to be genuinely more loving to myself and even to him.

[PARTNER]

Here he was crying, pleading with me to stay, to not leave. He did appear to be sincere. I believed him in the moment, but I had heard some of this before. The counselor told me that he believed him. I thought the counselor was telling me I was supposed to forgive him. But I needed time. I needed to see different action. I will say my anger has quieted. For now I stay focused on what I need to do for me, knowing that it will be of help to us recreating a different relationship. As for forgiveness—I think I love him, and there are things I respect about him, but I will just see where this healing journey leads me.

SELF-FORGIVENESS

In addition to forgiving your partner, you need to look at forgiving yourself for any behavior that has hurt others and your behavior that has hurt you. You may have been unavailable to your children or close friends because you were caught up in the throes of preoccupation or depression. You may have had a revenge affair or hurt yourself with negative self-talk. You may have lied and covered up for the addict. You need to forgive yourself for ignoring your suspicions, for making unfair comparisons by idealizing his lover and degrading yourself, for discounting your own perceptions, for tolerating the abusive behavior, and for making peace at any cost. The list can seem endless. You are human and you deserve acceptance for who you are in your humanness.

[JACQUE]

Even more helpful to me in my recovery than coming to forgive my husband was coming to forgive myself. I have been able to forgive myself for my sexual acting out, for how my fears allowed me to stay a doormat and not be confrontational, for how I would back down from my ultimatums, and for how I would berate myself and doubt myself. Oh, I had beaten myself up so much of my life. It is nice to get to a place where I don't do that anymore and, even more so, have incredible compassion for why and how I did those things to myself.

To get to a place of self-forgiveness you begin by stopping your negative self-talk, such as "I should have known better, I'm so stupid." You aren't stupid; you shouldn't have known better. Self-recrimination will only make you feel worse. You were scared, operating from a place of low esteem; you may simply have not known how to protect yourself, honor yourself, or express your feelings any differently. It's so much easier for women to extend compassion to others than to themselves. So pause, be reflective, and extend that courtesy to yourself. Self-forgiveness comes by taking baby steps; it doesn't come all at once, but you too can get to this place of self-love that other women have gotten to.

[PARTNER]

I have had to forgive myself for a lot of my behavior that was hurtful toward myself. A biggie for me was that I felt like I prostituted myself to him in doing sexual things I didn't want to do just to keep him happy or to keep him from getting angry. Today I accept that that behavior came from being scared, not having a strong sense of my own worth. I don't want to ever be in that place again.

[VANESSA]

I cannot stress enough how important the concepts of self-forgiveness and self-love were to me. Until I truly forgave and loved myself, I had no capacity to give the same gift to someone else.

With forgiveness you can look at your partner apart from his behavior and weigh the good and the bad. You can look with empathy toward yourself and how you contributed to the impairment in the relationship. You can give up the need for revenge, stop obsessing about what has occurred, and reengage in your own life.

[PARTNER]

Forgiveness took time—time for me to heal; to come to my own rescue; to sort out all the confusion, control, and obsession; and to let go. It also took the help of a counselor. For me, forgiveness had many prongs. I had to forgive my parents, my abuser, my husband, and most importantly I had to forgive myself. Forgive myself for not being perfect, for not protecting myself, for not getting help and into recovery sooner.

For you to heal it is necessary to have a commitment to healing; forgiveness will then take care of itself. Forgiveness is something that you come to gradually over time in degrees. Ultimately, it is your own powerful spirit that will heal you.

Spirituality: Where Is Your God?

Infidelity and all that comes with it doesn't leave you much time or energy for the emotional work required to build or maintain a connection with God or a Higher Power. You may not be the least bit convinced that a spiritual solution is the answer. You may have little practice in allowing God into your life, or you may be questioning your faith. So how does spirituality fit into this picture? Consider the fact that the problems you are facing may be so debilitating that human power alone is not sufficient to handle them.

It's possible your entire life has been about reacting, surviving, and keeping vigilant watch over outside forces. You've found your esteem through others; you've been trying to please, accommodate, and take care of others. However, discovering your true self cannot be done solely from the outside. Healing changes the course of your search for serenity from the outer world to the inner world.

When you know you can take care of yourself, and when you know you have the inner resources to make it, you do not have to live in hypervigilance any longer. You can say no to your shame. By doing these things, you move beyond the confines of the past on a course of spirituality in the present. As this happens, you will realize you cannot rely on your partner to make you whole, and you can and will be okay with or without him.

You deserve the opportunity to make that inward journey. In *A Dialogue with Hasidic Tales,* Maurice Friedman relates the Hasidic belief that if you want to change from one reality to another, you must first go through a "between-stage" in which you must morph into a blank slate. During this between-stage you will experience a "holy despair," which happens when you know that no other help will come except that which is from a Higher Power. When you accept that you cannot be the Higher Power yourself, it is the turning point of your recovery. When you come to believe that the Higher Power is all around you and also within you, that marks the turning point of your spirituality.[2]

[JACQUE]

My spirituality was compartmentalized. Like the rest of my life: broken, separate, not flowing. I grew up Catholic, went to church, and followed the rules, but it was something I had to do. Prayer offered me no solace. They were just words to repeat. The weekend my husband told me he was leaving was the weekend of Easter. I felt as if I were in a slimy pit with slick walls and no way to climb to the top. I was truly alone with no one to tell, no one to talk to. I listened through my pain to the inner voice that said, "Go to Mass." I hauled myself off to church and cried through the entire service. I'm sure the priest thought I was nuts. It may sound funny, but I could feel the presence of God, perhaps for the first time in my life. I think I was so raw, so empty, I had finally hit bottom and there was an opening in my armor to allow God into my life. I had let go because I felt I had hit a wall; there was nothing left. By finally finding God, I had an ability to turn my life and will over.

The Serenity Prayer has become so valuable to me.

Sometimes I journal and use each line of the prayer as a starting point. It helps me sort out, sift through, and give up to God. I love my God Box, too. Whenever I am struggling with an issue, thought, or obsession, I write it down and put it in the box. It actively helps me let go, and it works! I know God is present; I can hear and I can listen. A therapist once asked me where I thought God was when I was being abused as a child. At first I said clearly God was not around. But really when I think about it, God can't stop the evil in the world. He must have been present. I'm still alive, fairly normal, and not mentally insane. He protected my spirit, kept me whole, and led me to recovery. God had to have been there protecting me and my psyche.

Spirituality for me is different from going to church.

For me, spirituality is finding God in the everyday world around me: in nature, in the breath of wind, in my dog's smile. I look to God when I get cut off in traffic and say, "Oh well, God must not want me to get there now." And I used to have road rage! Obviously, I had a lot of anger, and the only place I felt safe getting it out was raging at other faceless, nameless drivers around me.

I have learned to pray about anything and everything, to seek God's guidance, and, more importantly, to thank God for my life.

Most partners I work with, such as Jacque, come to find acceptance and peace in their lives as they embrace a God or a Higher Power. Some women exercise faith in a Higher Being through their religious practice or at their house of worship; others find theirs through their twelve-step involvement.

[MAITE]

Before recovery, my spiritual life was about a God out there whom I had to please in order to be loved—a lot like my relationship with my parents. Since recovery, I've learned about other spiritual practices, especially Zen Buddhism. I meditate several times a day, I trust my inner guidance, and I am learning to let my husband and kids trust theirs. I look for the sacred in everything, especially inside myself and in others.

[SARA]

My ingrained religious practices just weren't working; they were too judgmental, too fear-based, and involved too much magical thinking. My religion was more about having a formula; if you do A-B-C, then D will happen. But it doesn't work that way. It was in twelve-step programs that I learned spiritual principles, such as showing up, service, and unconditional love. In Al-Anon, I would show up and not talk. I couldn't talk because the pain was too great. I went for months and months. They welcomed me. They supported me. I felt the love. I had never in my life felt unconditional love. What I was learning gave me a chance to live in the present—spirituality was freedom, a bigger plan that was not up to me to control. And I desperately needed something I wasn't trying to control. This spiritual path worked. There's a twelve-step saying, "It works if you work it," and I just did my best to work it even when I was totally skeptical, which I was.

My inner knowing is my best companion. I don't have to deny it, hide it, or explain it to be able to fit into any intellectual or religious group, as I did before. Today I think of addiction as a privileged journey of losses, pain, fear, and grieving to teach me to let go of my attachments to outside persons and things, and to go into my soul in order to find my wholeness and my divine. It is the universal connection to everything and everybody. That is the gift.

Sara was learning what Gary Zukav, author of *The Seat of the Soul*, says: "Your soul is not a passive or theoretical entity that occupies a space in the vicinity of your chest cavity. It is a positive purposeful force at the core of your being."[3]

[JENNY]

My faith saved me. I hurled myself into reading scripture and listening to sermons and Christian music on the radio. I joined recovery Bible studies. All of this gave me the courage and a foundation to come out of denial and into reality. I came to realize that instead of asking for what I needed and wanted, I was covertly trying to manipulate others to get what I wanted. As soon as I confessed that I had been trying to control the situations and the people in my household, God was faithful to give me strength to trust Him. Every time things worked out fine! God revealed to me that feelings of unworthiness separate us from Christ. I had to accept all of myself before I could let Christ accept me. I had to find out that there was a part of myself that I was denying.

[PARTNER]

I feel several things from my culture are helpful and they are closely related to my Catholic/African-Indigenous mix. The most important one is having faith in a universal Higher Power that is in charge of everything. I am not alone. There are guiding beings, seen and unseen, often help me when I need it. I know the pain and darkness are not forever. They are only challenges that make me stronger as a person and purify my soul. With patience (Let Go) and faith (Let God), everything is possible.

[VANESSA]

The key for me was moving from my rigid religious upbringing to an authentic relationship with a loving God. I have studied Jesus, Buddha, shamans, and saints, and have come to believe that a true connection to your Divine is paramount to your journey. It was about finding quiet in my soul and learning the gifts of "being" in all circumstances. Self-love, forgiveness, peace, and equanimity are all keys to healing that I can only find when this part of my soul has been ignited. To me, surrender is impossible without God. Releasing my pain was only possible when I had a powerful, loving God to give it to. That represented true healing to me. I no longer deny or hold on to my pain because I now believe that something greater than me will look after it. I truly connected with my Divine by working through years of religious indoctrination to establish a connection within myself and my God. This allowed me to find the powerful gifts of surrender and forgiveness, which has resulted in peace. To genuinely resonate with peace and love in my soul was a path to healing.

Even if you don't come from a background where you were introduced to a Higher Power or you do not have a history connected to a specific faith, be open to the possibility. These women found incredible direction and peace in their spiritual practice.

THE SPIRITUAL PATH

For a path to enhance the evolution of your spiritual well-being, it must be creative, not destructive; progressive, not regressive. It must stimulate and enhance, not stifle your spiritual well-being. In *The Teachings of Don Juan*, Carlos Castaneda writes, "Look at every path closely and deliberately. Try it as many times as you feel is necessary. Then ask yourself, and yourself alone, one question: Does this path have a heart? If it does, it is good; if it doesn't then it is of no use."[4]

Many women in recovery develop a spiritual path in their relationship to nature, song, or meditation. Julia Cameron, author of *The Artist's Way*, has instructed millions of women on the practice of daily morning free writing, which she calls Morning Pages.[5] Daily free writing or journaling can be grounding, centering, and a wonderful form of meditation. Other contemplative pursuits, such as physical activity, singing, and connecting to nature, will also still and free your mind.

[JACQUE]

Walking has become my time of contemplation. In my walking I find silence. I find beauty in my path. There is a stillness in which I go within.

[PARTNER]

Bicycling has been the time I feel a physical and personal strength, and in that time I am able to feel my feelings and gain a sense of direction. I take these wonderful moments in my ride to stop in some incredible scenic places and just be still.

Think about meditation literally. Many women in their fear and anger have metaphorically developed hardened or closed hearts. The closed heart cuts off the flow of the blood to itself and other body parts. The clinical term for this is *atherosclerosis*, a process by which plaque builds up and interferes with the flow of the coronary arteries. Famed heart specialist Dr. Dean Ornish, in his studies in India, recognized the connection between unresolved anger and fear (closed heart chakra and closed coronary arteries) and found that diet, exercise, support groups, and meditation could reverse heart disease without invasive procedures.[6] In many languages, cognates of the word *spirit* mean *breath* or *to breathe*. Meditation allows you to open your heart and lungs. It offers the opportunity to clear your mind and be present with the here and now. It doesn't matter which spiritual path you take (Christianity, Judaism, Islam, Mother Earth, or others) or what form it takes (prayer, song, nature, meditation), what's important is that you keep moving forward and growing on the path you have chosen.

Questions you may want to consider:

- If you practice a particular faith, how can it support you in your healing process?

- If you have no specific faith or religion, what spiritual practice might you try?

- What form of spiritual practice appeals to you? Are you willing to try it?

- Do you find sound or silence conducive to a sense of spiritual connection?

- Have you established, or could you establish, any personal daily rituals?

Author Brian Seaward, in his book *Stand Like Mountain, Flow Like Water*, speaks of the path using the metaphor of a mountain climber seeking the summit. He says, "To stand on a mountain peak epitomizes the expression 'I have touched the face of God.' Yet the trip of life doesn't end at the mountaintop. One only stays long enough to enjoy the view and become inspired before beginning the descent. There is no one best route up the mountain, only several paths each offering different experiences." He goes on to quote author Glen Clark: "If you wish to travel far and fast, travel light. Take off all of your envies, jealousies, unforgiveness, selfishness, and fears."[7]

There are no porters on the spiritual path; you have to carry your own baggage. The ultimate question in addressing spiritual growth becomes, *How can I best nurture a relationship with a Higher Power?*

As a woman, you may feel that society often expects you to operate at a higher ground; you are supposed to be understanding, forgiving, and spiritual. In an attempt to be a "good" woman you try to skip over the emotional work and go directly to the spiritual realm. Or you attempt to find inner peace and harmony from an intellectual understanding, or you throw yourself into volunteer work to demonstrate your spiritual intent. While any sincere effort can be extremely valuable, you cannot singularly will yourself to a higher plane. You cannot skip any steps. You cannot be a spiritual person unless you apply yourself to the necessary work. To grow spiritually you must walk the walk.

Practicing spirituality means that you:

- Do the footwork.

- Are present, being in the here and now.

- Stay attuned to your inner guidance.

- Be authentic.

- Put forth the effort.

- Let go of the attachment to the results.

- Believe in divine guidance and the choice it offers.

- Engage regularly and repetitively.

As you grow spiritually, you will learn to trust that life will continue to unfold, as it must.

[SARA]

I practice staying in touch with a loving God on a daily basis. It begins in the morning for me with a meditation reading from one of those many day-by-day meditation books. My God is a loving, not punishing God. I believe the more love you feel toward others is the essence of God. Accept people for who they are with their imperfections—now that doesn't mean sacrificing myself to a victim role, but that means letting go of judgment of both others and myself and loving myself with healthy boundaries.

Your spirituality acknowledges and does homage to the spark of divinity within you; it is an approach to life, an attitude. When lived, practiced consistently, and acted on consciously, it reinforces your commitment to personal transformation. This manifests itself most clearly in your attitude toward life. Your personal spirituality is a blend of your purposeful intent to be authentic and trust your intuition. Authenticity and intuition are hallmarks of your recovery. From this foundation follows a willingness to continue learning from life.

"I cannot separate what I conceive as Spirit from my concept of God.

Thus I believe that God is Spirit."

Maya Angelou

Reflective Thoughts and Questions

- What does forgiveness mean to you?

- Do you think you have engaged in cheap or false forgiveness?

- Have you forgiven yourself?

- Is faith or a belief in a Higher Power an important part of your life today? If so, describe.

- Is spirituality an aspect of your life you are willing to explore more as it relates to your recovery process?

- What was important for you to learn in this chapter?

CHAPTER EIGHT NOTES

1   Janis Spring with Michael Spring, *How Can I Forgive You? The Courage to Forgive, the Freedom Not To* (New York: HarperCollins, 2004).

2   Maurice Friedman, *A Dialogue with Hasidic Tales* (New York: Human Science Press, 1988).

3   Gary Zukav, *The Seat of the Soul* (New York: Fireside, 1989) 31

4   Carlos Castaneda, *The Teachings of Don Juan: A Yaqui Way of Knowledge* (New York: Washington Square Press, 1985) 82.

5   Julia Cameron, *The Artist's Way: A Spiritual Path to Higher Creativity* (New York: J. P. Tarcher/Putnam, 2002).

6   Dean Ornish, *Dr. Dean Ornish's Program for Reversing Heart Disease* (New York: Random House, 1990).

7   Brian Seaward, *Stand Like Mountain, Flow Like Water* (Deerfield Beach, FL: Health Communications, Inc., 1997), 56–7.

CHAPTER NINE

The Women of the Lodge

Change takes time. Recovery is a process.

Trust and give voice to your reality.

Begin your healing journey.

Living in a society of instant gratification, with instant access to a world of information and transactions in the palm of your hand, it's easy to show up at a therapist's office or twelve-step meeting and expect an instant solution to all of the problems that come from living with sex addiction. But recovery is a process, not an event. It is a process with no guarantees about the relationship, but a process that does guarantee a journey to self-love and self-care.

You no longer have to tolerate the hurtful. You can trust your own perceptions and give voice to your reality. You can move forward in truth. Secrets disappear and the potential for connectedness with self, others, and the universe is fully there. You deserve to continue your life free of fear, confusion, denial, and shame. You deserve to believe in your preciousness and to have it honored from within and by those you invite into your life. This is possible when you allow others to be a part of your process, as did the Women of the Lodge. These women found a path; they have tools and they have faith. Let's continue with their stories and see how their journeys have progressed.

[THERESE]

Why would I need my own recovery? After all, he had the problem. Now I just shake my head at my thinking I was so much better than him. Recovery has been my life blessing.

I certainly knew that my husband needed help, but I've had a hard time realizing that I needed help too. I believed I was entitled to say and do whatever I wanted. After all, I was the victim. When he started his recovery, I wanted him to change but I found that I was jealous about him giving his time to his recovery. I actually became more obsessive about whether or not he was on the internet once he was in recovery. I was shameless in my sleuth work trying to trap him. He seemed to feel better about himself, but I actually became angrier. I was interpreting everything to be about me. He owed me now. What was he going to do for me? What was he going to do to assure me that he wasn't going to look at other women? I wasn't giving him any support, although periodically for the sake of being nice.

I would go to one of his therapy sessions. I did not want to talk in front of those people. I had nothing to say to them. Then things began to crumble even more when our fourteen-year-old got into trouble with drugs and sex. I thought we were going to lose her. One night she was almost raped. I also knew that my husband was in a serious relapse. I drove myself to see his counselor. As much as I had set out to catch him in a relapse, when he actually had one I let go of my entire ego. For the first time I realized I didn't have the answers and I was a mess.

I was so scared and numb I simply did what his counselor told me and showed up at a group with other women. For several weeks I didn't talk, I just cried quietly. They gently accepted me, my tears, and my silence. I so respected these women; they were angry, they cried, they laughed. Feelings were everywhere, and yet they could talk about them. Slowly I began to talk about myself.

They wouldn't let me talk about my husband. I came to really understand that his behavior was not about me. I heard that early on but didn't truly understand it. Pornography was his answer to his fears; it was his fix and it became addictive. My issue is my lack of a strong sense of knowing myself, deriving my self-esteem from how we looked, and having control over my feelings but not being honest about them.

Today I work hard at recognizing and talking about my feelings. I'm aware when I mask them and can even laugh at myself for how readily I use my defenses. I don't think I can say I like showing my vulnerability but I do it. And of all the people, it is my husband who most understands and accepts me. When I show him this part of me he meets me where I am. Mostly I get scared. I get scared of the unknown more than anything real. So I work a lot at staying in the here and now. I don't schedule all of my time or the family's time.

And after months now, I can say it works. I have time to be spontaneous, to be available to others, to listen to myself. I am not running from myself anymore. And better yet, I like myself more. I like my husband more. I like life more.

I realize I have been scared a lot of my life—certainly long before my marriage started. Mostly I have been scared that I'm not good enough. I always acted like I was above everyone else and separate from them. By the time I got to my first group I was so humbled. I felt like I was crawling out from some deep hole in the ground. Maybe others didn't see this superiority of mine, but I knew I had been hiding behind it all of my life.

Today I am proud, truly proud to be accepting and available to all the women as they come through the doors of the Lodge. As different as we are, our underbellies are the same. I have been in group with a lot of different women and I have very strong friendships with some of them. I respect all of them for just showing up. I know how hard that is. Recovery is very humbling.

In the long run I don't know what all of this means for my marriage, but I'm hopeful. I know that being quietly angry and playing the martyr is not going to make our marriage work, and I already feel so much better about myself, him, and us.

When your partner uses pornography to act out, as Therese's did, it is common to rationalize that your situation is very different from others whose partners' acting out involves flesh-and-blood people. Whether it's pornography, cybersex, or other behaviors such as voyeurism or exhibitionism that don't involve actual bodily contact with others, the process of holding yourself apart and different only increases the likelihood that you will miss the opportunity to heal from your pain. Or you could miss the opportunity to join your partner in a coupleship based on mutual healing and recovery, as Therese almost did. While Therese came slowly to the realization that there were an incredible number of gifts for her in the recovery process, she also came to realize she had fewer differences and much more in common with the other Women of the Lodge than she anticipated.

[VANESSA]

When I first found out my husband had exposed me to chlamydia while I was pregnant, I took his minimal disclosure as yet another call to action in my life. Let's just buckle down and fix this. We both entered our respective twelve-step programs and therapy. I was happy to have some other cause to focus on, another project I could fix. This attitude changed approximately three months later when I found his First Step document. The level of infidelity detailed in it was shocking! I was enraged and I turned into this evil, vindictive woman bent on making him pay. The next few months were hell for both of us. I felt my life was crumbling. It was impossible to be the perfect wife, perfect mother, perfect work-addicted employee, and perfect friend to all the needy people I had surrounded myself with, while my foundational belief system was being shattered in every way. It was a crisis time in my life, and luckily I chose to look at my own stuff—my work addiction and issues—and make some changes. It was such a hard year but pivotal to my recovery. I quit my high-powered job, became a full-time mom, and dug into recovery in a serious way. My life was forever altered by that decision.

My don't talk/denial training was so ingrained I found it very difficult to share the dark side of my life with people. Twelve-step programs helped a lot because they were a safe place to share with others undergoing similar experiences and pain. Initially I found it very difficult to discuss this with my friends, partly because I had spent so much time selling my perfect life to myself and others. I had a new awareness of how emotionally shut down I was as I realized that, even though I had a ton of friends, I had become very proficient in becoming close to people by listening to all their problems and encouraging them to share their issues but disclosing very little about myself. It was a very big step for both me and my husband to come out. It was so important for me to start breaking my childhood rules—don't talk, don't feel—by telling on myself and becoming vulnerable with safe people.

In my recovery I did a lot of trauma work related to my childhood. I would come to confront my father about his raging behavior. The trauma work was so necessary as I struggled with slow leakage of disclosures as they dribbled out over a few years. I would let go of my need to be in control. I would let go of my perfectionism. I would embrace my beauty and that inner child who needed nurturing. I would learn to trust myself. My husband and I worked hard, not without relapse and pain. We were truly finding some happiness when another bomb dropped—I

was diagnosed with aggressive ovarian cancer.
Now this would be a true test of recovery.

I cannot tell you how valuable all those trite adages
of recovery became to me during this time: One
day at a time. Let go and let God. You're never
given more than you can handle. Those incredible
lessons became lifelines for me, and I became
vulnerable in a way I had never known. I was so
broken; I was truly fighting for my life. I finally
learned to reach out, to ask for help. In the darkest
time of my life, I actually found what it was like to
seize life. Looking at my son, I really understood
how important it was to seize every single moment.
I believe that recovery was instrumental in saving
my life because my physical death sentence
became a spiritual and emotional growth period.
In facing death, I became more alive. I believe my
husband walked with me on this journey. In an act
of solidarity he shaved his head so I wouldn't be
bald alone while I underwent chemotherapy. My
many friends supported us with vigils of prayer
and friendship before every major treatment,
whether it was surgery, chemo, or major testing.
He was there for every one of those, seemingly
invested in the whole process. But the Jekyll and
Hyde of addiction was clearly at play again. One
year after my diagnosis (and bleak prognosis), he
was called to come clean to me at an intensive
treatment center. Apparently the whole time he
was holding my hand through cancer, he was also
engaging in sexual relationships with escorts,
having affairs with other women, and soliciting
sexual relations with adventurous couples. As
I sat in the therapist's office listening to his full

disclosure, still bald from the chemo, I felt a part of me die inside. I had never felt such brokenness, such blatant and deceptive betrayal, in my darkest hour. It was then that I knew my recovery journey was far from over. I had some serious relationship/ recovery decisions to make.

Right or wrong—there can be no second guessing—I made the decision to stay. And though I labored over that choice with therapists, I realize looking back that I was simply not strong enough to leave at that time. I was only then starting to look at what drove me to be in such a hurtful relationship. Until I cleaned up the baggage in my soul, I would never be able to truly look at the dis-ease in our relationship. I was still operating inherently from that place of not good enough.

The good news is we both went to new levels of healing. Things seemingly smoothed out. Then another painful life event occurred. My sister, who had been in remission for many years, found out she was now dying of her cancer. She was in terrible pain and needed constant assistance. I faced my sister's death and my own mortality with a new level of healing.

Vanessa's situation speaks to comments I made in Chapter Two about factors that influence the depth of trauma. For Vanessa, in addition to chronic sexual betrayal, the types of behavior her husband engaged in exacerbated her trauma. Her childhood trauma and the trauma associated to her own health issues as well as being confronted with her sister dying all influenced the impact of her traumas. She found that she would benefit using a variety of trauma modalities to aid her in her healing.

Vanessa continues her recovery practices and in that process she grows emotionally and spiritually strong. She moves in and out of active cancer and remission. She is at a place of calm in her life and she is feeling strong in her marriage when, to her surprise, her husband decides to leave the marriage to be with another woman.

I wish that I could share with you a "happily ever after" ending that I spent most of my life fantasizing about.

Alas, though recovery has been one of the greatest gifts of my life, it did not have the ability to save my marriage. Addiction is cunning and baffling; it's a prickly thing that takes a lifelong commitment to avoid relapse. After seven years in recovery together, my husband went back out.

I pray for him as a human being and the father of my child. I have finally learned the meaning of letting go. It is through the hardships I have encountered in my life that I learned about the need to surrender, to live in the now, and to focus on me and a journey of self-love. I make a commitment daily to operate from a place of gratitude, authenticity, and congruency so that I can truly live life and strive to make a difference in this world.

Sadly, even with recovery practice, there are no promises of marital bliss. Vanessa's husband made various choices along his path and in his journey he wasn't honest with her about his feelings or his behavior. He made the choice to leave the marriage. Steeped in her recovery process, Vanessa would come to an inner peace, knowing that her recovery is not based on being in this marriage.

This journey of healing has been painful and arduous. It has also been so rewarding and life-changing. And it's far from over; recovery is a journey, not a destination. Every day I look into my soul for toxic messages and unhealthy behaviors. Every day I look for the beauty in every moment, for the joys of my relationships, and for the gifts of my recovery. I live the paradoxes. My spiritual and emotional paths are so rich and authentic. I talk, I feel, and I love. I know that this is yet another step on my journey and that I have lots more to learn. I also know there is no happily ever after, but there can be peace and joy in the moment. And now is all we really have.

As a woman who strongly identifies with her culture, Maite has chosen to confront the rules of silence that fuel addiction as well as the societal rules of being a Latina. With the support of other women, she embraces a newfound freedom to let go of social and familial constraints and find intimacy with herself and her husband.

[MAITE]

I have found I need support and I need therapy, not as a punishment for his behaviors but as a way of understanding and healing. I deserve recovery, too. I spent a lot of years in my good/perfect/saint role: someone who saw herself as better than my husband in my saintly behavior. Like many Latinos and Latinas, I am a very proud person. But I see how this disease affects everyone involved. I see it affect coworkers, family members on both sides, and friends. It certainly affected me. It pains me to see women who don't want to be in recovery for themselves, who choose to hang on to that false pride, who prefer to stay in the "better than" thinking. Not for me, no longer.

Before recovery I had walls of fear to control and protect me from others. Today in my recovery I have the gift of knowing I don't need to control. In fact, by letting go of my controlling behaviors I have found a freedom I've never known. In that freedom I don't have to hide my fears or my shame; I feel love for myself and my husband. And I've learned about boundaries. I've discovered that boundaries are about honoring and respecting me and others physically, emotionally, intellectually—the spiritual sacred spaces—living honestly and with integrity.

In my family and in my culture, everyone is into everyone else's business. I was trained never to question authorities or loved ones, even when my intellect or my intuition knew my truth. Enmeshment brings a lot of abuse. If someone has a pain, I am supposed to cry. If you have a need, I am to meet it. If you are fat, I am to be fat. If a neighbor is sad, I am supposed to be in mourning too. That is no longer okay with me. Today I am learning I have the right to say no, I have the right to my own feelings, I don't have to caretake to be a good human being.

I am fortunate because my husband wants recovery.

He doesn't want to keep living his secret life. But I know I can have my recovery with or without him. I am no longer willing to live with the dishonesty, the lying, and the craziness where I doubt myself when the truth is not spoken. Now my healthy self knows what it knows and I honor it. It doesn't matter who gets upset.

My husband is a businessman and many people know us. I used to participate in everything. People in our community, people in our family, and people in other families asked us for all kinds of help, from money to jobs to assistance with visa paperwork for new immigrant families. I used to give money, time, write letters, and lots of things to anyone when asked. Now I say no when I want to. I don't think I have to do what they want in order for me to be a good person. I know I am a good person. We have a good, economical life so I thought I was obligated to caretake our many family members, friends, and employees. I gave and gave and gave, and it was never enough. I felt guilty, angry, and used. Now I choose. Today I find myself saying no to anything that interferes with my spiritual life, my interior life.

Today I have much laughter in my life. By not trying to control and manipulate everything and everyone, and by not being vigilant about the rules of perfection, it's so much easier to find the laughter and humor in everyday life. Laughter gives me a freedom to be myself, to know my feelings, to be imperfect, to let go of judgment, to find serenity. I don't live a role anymore. I wear fun, colorful clothes. At times I know my kids might prefer I be a bit less colorful, but I simply find humor in that as well.

My kids have the typical young adult challenges, but my recovery tools have made me a better mother.

In addition to being with other women in recovery groups, I make a point of socializing with some of them outside of group. We go to movies, we go to the mall, we have coffee, and we spend a lot of that time laughing. I don't live all bound up in other people's expectations—my husband's, my family's, or my culture. I have come to a place in my recovery where I love myself. I nurture my body, my spirit, and our relationship. As difficult as reality can be and as frightening as honesty sometimes is, living in truth has been so freeing. As for what happens in my marriage, for now we each practice our recovery. Learning to communicate has been vital and at times still awkward. I think I sometimes overwhelm my husband with my openness. I'm sure that it's shocking, given that early in our marriage I learned to be very silent. There is no hiding from each other. I trust that whatever it is, if we talk about it, it will be okay. When I feel like I just want to attack him, I ask myself, "What are my intentions?" Healthy intention is not to make him feel bad, not to control or manipulate, but to seek the truth. The truth is the path to healing. Living in reality is necessary. He is a mirror of my reality; when he lies or just doesn't tell me something then the reality gets distorted. I am not preoccupied with his recovery, but I know he has to be in recovery for us to be a couple. We love each other no matter how sick we are, but we need to heal this sickness.

We are not the perfect family; perfect is an illusion, perfect is crushed, and perfect is not real. The fairy tale is not there. Today we are a family—a family with a lot of love and a lot of good communication.

After years of seeking the help of multiple therapists who basically told her the problem was in her head, Maite challenged the gender and cultural teachings that had been so strongly ingrained into her being: your needs are not important, discount your perceptions, defer to the man, don't question, look good at all costs, never complain. This was quite a fight for her, but while waging it she found a path that led to self-love, self-care, and true joy by living in the truth. And in that process, her husband joined her in the journey.

[JACQUE]

When my husband and I finally named what was happening in our lives, I wanted to know everything there was to know about sex addiction and what to do about it. I wanted it all tied up in a neat little box so I could have control of my life again. I wanted a promise that we would work it out. I wanted recovery for us, not so much for me. Little did I know that what I really needed was to let go completely and give it all up to see what would come back to me. I would ultimately need to walk through my life with a sifter to bring the fine and delicate pieces of my life back together and to toss away the chunks that really didn't work for me (the control, resentment, anger, fear, lack of trust, and misplaced trust) no matter how much I hung on to them. I felt so broken I wanted to be with others who maybe knew how it was, if that was possible.

I found other women who had walked in similar shoes. I listened and began to talk about my experiences. I had so much shame about my behavior, our behavior, and my husband's behavior. But I felt such acceptance and love from these other women. I wanted what I saw some of them had: a voice. They could talk about their feelings. They had a sense of how to take care of themselves. They were struggling for sure, not knowing what was totally real in their own relationships, confused about whether or not to go or stay, and angry about the betrayal, the consequences. Together we would heal. I had a lot to learn about the power of being with other women and how to be good to myself in a nurturing way.

In spite of the incredible struggle to confront and change old beliefs and behaviors, I discovered so much about me. But I can't say it came easy. My insides often screamed in protest of what I had to let go of to get to a greater place of wholeness. I discovered the only way to trust again was to learn to trust myself. I learned to be honest in all areas of my life. I learned nothing could ever be the same again. All of my interactions would be different because I was different. I learned to let go completely, to trust in God. I learned the power of supportive women in my life. I learned to trust women. I learned to speak up for myself in an empowering way. I learned to share the hard stuff: the pain, fear, anger, and resentments. I learned to tell on myself, my mistakes and fears. I learned the power of laughter and fun. I learned to listen. I learned to honor myself as a woman; to hold on to that and never let it go. I learned I am controlling and judgmental, not perfect. I learned to honor that part of me too. I learned to trust therapy. I learned I couldn't do it on my own, no matter how hard I tried. I needed the group. I needed a sponsor, and I needed friends.

Much of my recovery has come from being willing to talk about the sex abuse in my childhood, from grieving the loss that came with not being able to have children, and from breaking my denial about how men have chronically abused me. I have worked to transition from sex abuse victim to survivor. I read numerous books, but one in particular, called *The Courage to Heal*, spoke to me, and I spent the next year working the exercises. I felt such shame the day I purchased it. I wanted to hide it and pretend I was buying it for someone else. Then I told my parents about the sexual abuse my brother performed on me. I have no real memory of the time frame other than knowing about when it started and about when it ended, somewhere about five years. I do have some specific memories, and through my recovery I have discovered I have a very strong case of post-traumatic stress disorder related to the abuse. I also used the incredible therapy tool of Eye Movement Desensitization Reprocessing (EMDR) to lessen my anxiety and reframe loving beliefs about myself as well as allowing myself to be heard, allowing myself a voice, allowing myself to grieve, and then to be held safely by wonderfully caring women.

I learned to "do" recovery, to have a plan as to what my recovery could look like. I was looking at me and not living in reactivity to my husband. I would go to meetings and share. I found the courage and support to start my own twelve-step group for partners since I lived in an area where there were no groups. I learned that I am a part of the whole, that my part is just as important as any other woman in the group. I feel whole and believe in myself.

I quit feeling less than, and I stopped comparing myself to others: I stopped competing. I have begun to use the other half of my brain, to allow my artistic side to rise to the surface, to let what was there flow in the way it was intended. I listen and accept feedback. I discern what will and will not work for me. I've stopped defending myself, stopped giving my power away, and stopped giving myself away. I hold myself as precious. I experience the power of women, the power of tradition and ceremony.

I have had to get therapy to help me get to a place of healthy anger. I have ripped up my share of Kleenex. I have beaten the bed. I also kick things, and I walk hard, and I air box. I have a great time with my anger and it's empowering. But having been a major peacekeeper in my life, I can still go there when I get scared. And my husband's anger can scare me. So I always work at boundaries, knowing whose stuff is whose. I don't take on his blaming. I am not willing to be abused. Today I recognize it early on and I have learned to stick up for myself verbally and remove myself from the situation if that is necessary.

My best boundary is in knowing I cannot do his recovery. Today in his work he still travels some so I talk about any fears I have. I no longer bury my head in the sand. If he chooses not to follow his recovery plan, then I really believe it will be a short amount of time and I will know. And then I am free to make my own decisions. Today I stay because I feel hope for us. I feel hope because I see a change in behavior. We communicate so much better and so much more than before. I am more trusting of myself with him, more willing to be genuinely vulnerable and he so with me. Today I have learned to ask for assistance to allow people to be of support.

In the early stages of our relationship I had this desperate need not to be abandoned. The love I had for him morphed into not wanting to be alone. As we moved into our recovery and I began to value myself, to get my own esteem. I knew I didn't want to be in a relationship if he could not be present with me. I do remember what it was like to love him with all my heart and want to be with the kind, loving, fun man. And as he got working more and more on his recovery, I know this man is a man I do want to be with; he's kind, caring, fun, adventuresome. I was wounded long before I met my husband and he was the product of woundedness before his sex addiction. We are two wounded people tapping into our strengths and learning to be in this world in a way we never were before.

Jacque has worked hard in her recovery and, as you have just read, she talks about herself more than she talks about her marriage or her husband. This is what she takes to her marriage now, her recovery. With two therapeutic separations behind them, she and her husband are together and both of them are actively engaged in their recovery processes.

[JENNY]

For so many years I lived in denial and fantasy, beginning my marriage with a façade of seeing myself as righteous, capable, and having the world by the tail, yet having an inner world of self-loathing, terror, and confusion. After fifteen years of marriage and my husband acting out his many addictions, I was operating at a minimal level, experiencing severe depression and two nervous breakdowns. It was at this time that I began to seek my spirituality in Jesus. I prayed and prayed for my circumstances to change, but it wasn't until I took the Lord at His word that things did start to change! "There is none righteous, no, not one." I guess that meant me, but I thought I was so much better than my husband. "Take the log out of your own eye before you try to remove the speck from your brother's." Wow! It was *me* who I needed to ask the Lord to change!

This was hard. I saw myself totally as the victim and he an abuser. I began to be present with my prayer and came to realize that I had things I needed to address about myself. The style of my prayers changed. I asked for direction. I asked for courage and strength.

A few years into my spiritual journey, when I started to pray, "Lord change me," is when my husband actually began to change. At first his acting out became worse. Finally after a heartfelt disclosure he started looking for treatment centers. At this time I knew nothing about sex addiction. I was so naive that I didn't even know what a treatment center was. He said he was going for his drug addiction, but he took painstaking steps to pick out just the right one, and today I believe it is because he knew his sexual acting out was controlling him and severely hurting his family.

At the encouragement of the treatment program staff, I began therapy with a specialist in sex addiction so I could focus on my trauma issues. I didn't know what was wrong with me or even what had happened to me in my life, but I was willing to look at anything in my life that needed changing, *anything*. The scriptures told me, "Know the truth and the truth shall set you free." I knew I wanted to be free but I wasn't sure what I wanted to be freed from. I just knew I wanted to get out of the hell that I had been living in.

I would discover the shameful self that I had been trained to cover up and eventually forgot was there. It was buried alive, always nagging to come out, and actually coming out sideways in everything I did: how I related to my children, what I thought and felt about myself, and how I related to my husband. Judgment, condemnation, and control oozed from the pores in my skin.

I was working with a therapist to address my childhood history and my addiction to a sex addict. That is when I joined a support group at my church with other women whose partners acted out sexually. I also joined a codependency group at my church. The individual therapy would keep my head above water. It was in group I felt the validation I needed to move from a victim mentality, a childlike person, to trusting myself and asking for what I needed. It was in group that

I would learn how to connect with other people and not be so afraid of them.

I have no doubt that the single most powerful tool I had in my healing was my support groups. Without those women I could have never experienced the love and acceptance that Jesus wanted me to experience. I had never been comfortable in groups and didn't make friends easily. I was afraid of people, especially women. But in the group I learned to trust safe people; I learned to tell my story. I learned to confront my husband and I learned to tell him what I wanted and needed. I acquired incredible courage and conviction. As I healed spiritually I began to heal emotionally and relationally as well.

Then I was led to another group where I would go deeper into my recovery process and I could be more explicit about my abuse and my marriage. It was here I would work a lot on how much I was dissociating, not able to stay present. This had been going on for years. It was here I allowed myself to be seen, meaning I was able to share the self-loathing I often felt. And it would be in this group that I would become open enough to receive from others, to receive their caring, and with that, to come to really accept my worth. This healing process was essential for me because it helped me shatter the toxic shame that I carried. One of the more profound experiences I had in this group was that no matter what I had to say about what I had done or about what had been done to me, I experienced a sense of unconditional love and acceptance. The facilitators would guide me to look deeply into the eyes of each group member.

They'd have me hold that gaze for a significant amount of time before looking to the next person. This process helped to turn the lies that caused me self-hatred and shame into the truth of acceptance and my true value given to me by my Creator.

I would come to realize that my healing was the most important thing in my life, and to believe that my husband was standing in the way of my being able to fully heal. I decided I could not be with such a controlling and fearful husband. I wasn't strong enough to survive that, and I was committed to my healing. I really didn't know how I could support myself. I had not worked outside of the home in years. But I put one foot in front of the other, I prayed, and I was practical. After a couple years in recovery, as scary and financially difficult as it was, I chose to divorce. I didn't see my husband's recovery behavior as consistent with mine, and our differences were too great. I am not very confident in myself when it comes to relationships today, but I think that will pass. I know I am still fragile. But today I also feel my strength. I am grateful for what I have with my children; I recognize that I am smart. I am learning how to have fun, how to take care of me, and how to know and honor my feelings. Each day I feel stronger within.

I can actually feel my insides smile—this is a long way from my depression and nervous breakdowns.

Ultimately, Jenny's faith led her into a recovery process, and as she said, it gave her "the courage and foundation to come out of denial and into reality." She was readily able to embrace how the teachings of the Bible, together with her therapy process, offered a path to healing. Like many partners, she prayed, bargained, and pleaded with her God, and in time Jenny heard and listened. She approached therapy willingly, she followed direction, and she read all she could find about codependency and trauma. As scared as she was of allowing herself to open up to other women, she came to blossom in their strength and support.

[SARA]

Sara came into betrayal recovery after several years in Al-Anon. It is very likely her participation in a twelve-step program led her to trust in the group process and believe in the power of sharing with others with similar experiences.

I came to this group to meet other women with husbands who were acting out. I was so angry—angry that this is where I was in my life. I was not sure what I was hoping for. I had one foot ready to head out of this marriage, yet I came and am forever grateful for that.

Today when I think about my recovery, I see it so far in three levels. My first level began in Al-Anon; that was the beginning of my path. My husband had just gotten sober, but I was having trouble sleeping and eating, I was worried about money, and the kids were acting out. There wasn't a corner of my life that was peaceful. The concept of being responsible for the results of my own life despite what happens to me was a beginning, a big beginning.

The second level was the recovery more connected to sex addiction. Here again I was in crisis, not just from the knowledge my husband had been continuing to act out sexually and it was addictive, but I now had breast cancer. Also at this time three of my family members and friends passed away. While all levels of recovery begin with crisis, at this stage the crises were so much deeper, threatening, and terrifying. I needed to be led, supported, and comforted. I knew enough that I knew I couldn't do this alone. I sought out several professionals—counselors experienced in addressing codependency, sex addiction, and loss. I found medical help I trusted. Together they were my team; they helped me put one foot in front of the other. I was hurting and scared, and I needed to call upon every internal strength I had at a time of incredible brokenness. I listened to my host of guides, I followed direction, and I honored myself.

I had so much loss—loss of illusion, loss of health, loss of family and friends—and so much fear. I grieved and grieved, moving up and down and through all of the stages they talk about—anger, sadness, bargaining, guilt—sort of like in staccato fashion, with a lot of starts and stops. I would come to understand the generational repetitions in my family. This would offer me a framework to understand I wasn't crazy, I wasn't defective. I was simply wounded, and from that I could heal. I would put into practice healthy boundaries. I would learn to take down my walls and to be vulnerable but hold on to my integrity and esteem. I would also learn to listen and, more important, to hear. I learned better communication and problem-solving skills. I would constrain that part of me that wanted to lash out in my pain. I would also lighten up and not take myself so seriously all of the time. I practiced gratitude and laughter in my life a lot at this stage.

The third level of recovery, which would come within two to three years of beginning what I call level two, was to know myself differently than ever before. No matter what on earth happens to me, I will be all right. My being all right is not about his sobriety with alcohol or sex. I know I can get through whatever is there in front of me. I trust myself. Never again is it okay for someone to mistreat or abuse me. I realize when we first got together we were both desperately in love and saw ourselves as soul mates, star-crossed lovers. Then my love became conditional in the height of our addictions. Today I can say I love him, and I love him forever. Now that does not mean he can live with me forever. If he acts out and doesn't do anything about it that is mistreating me. I realize today I had my husband on a fairy-tale pedestal from the day we met; then, with his acting out, he crashed down from that pedestal. Today I am very aware of his faults and they can irritate me, but now I don't need him to be an illusion for me.

Being in recovery means every day belongs to me to express who I am in each thing I do. It means when I make the inevitable mistakes in that day, I have a way to set my conscience straight, no matter what the rest of the world says or thinks about my behavior. I know my heart and I know who and why I love. It is because of honesty and trust in my judgment and motives. I know my job is not to save anyone. I can't. I don't want to interfere with their beautiful but sometimes painful path. I do take great delight in being of loving service in this world. I sometimes quake in my boots from fear, but I know it can be shared with God and my trusted friends. I swirl and delight in the delicious joy and challenge of life. I play. I cry. I hurt. I laugh. I am beginning to trust that what I put out into the universe comes lovingly back to me. I am in partnership with those I choose, including my spouse. If any relationship becomes toxic for my well-being, I will be there for myself and take care of this precious life of mine.

People ask me how I live with knowing he could relapse. Well, there have been relapses and he could have more. I hope he doesn't. What I do know is that whatever comes about, it is not about me. His behavior is not about me. And I will handle whatever comes my way. Nothing is guaranteed.

When old habits and fears arise, there are friends whom I talk with through situations, disagreements, and challenges. Being in recovery means reaching out for this support when I feel myself lapsing back into the old patterns that made my life so miserable. My recovery friends are willing to call me on my stubbornness and control issues, or point out when I'm being self-righteous or self-centered.

The one area I think I have needed to stay most vigilant is my jumping to an emotional response. When I feel misunderstood or threatened, I go from neutral to an immediate fight-or-flight response. If we have a really heated argument, or worse, a disagreement that never gets expressed, my mind will quickly jump to thoughts of leaving and finding a more peaceful life. But I recognize that is old, fear-based behavior. Today I use my tools to work through feelings, to communicate, to own my needs, and to value them. We talk. We listen. We work toward the win-win.

My greatest strides have come with being with other women in recovery and twelve-step groups. It is a privilege to be able to go and tune up. The truth is what I recovered. I don't need to hide anymore.

As Sara said, she came to the Women of the Lodge group incredibly angry, but her Al-Anon experience had taught her that she would be safe with other women. In that safe environment she vented and ultimately owned her own shame and fears. She was able to make the connection and see how her early life abandonment was perpetuated in her adult relationships with men. The internal shift that propelled her life into one of laughter, connection, and peace occurred when she recognized that her healing was predicated on the commitment to no longer abandon herself.

The Invitation

The personal crises that Therese, Vanessa, Maite, Jacque, Jenny, and Sara experienced led them to pursue recovery specific to living with sex addiction. Therese began her journey a couple of years after her husband had begun his. Vanessa embraced recovery after being exposed to a sexually transmitted disease while she was pregnant. Just when Maite was ready to leave her marriage, she and her husband began their recovery journey. Jacque and her husband began their journey together as he was walking out the door to be with his girlfriend. Jenny began recovery when her husband sought treatment for his drug abuse and when his sexual behavior was also identified. Sara and her husband began theirs when she discovered a book on sex addiction in his car.

It may be discouraging to read about women who put their heart and soul into the healing and recovery process and still their relationship or marriage did not survive, as is true for two of the six women of the Lodge. Yet in spite of the present-day outcome of their relationships and what their partners did or didn't do in recovery, all of these women continue their healing journey. While their relationship problems got them into a recovery process, they stayed to heal themselves. This journey transcended the issues of betrayal and deceit and became one of personal healing never before imagined. They learned to trust their perceptions, listen to their feelings, recognize their needs, and establish respectful boundaries. They addressed their childhood trauma issues, recognized the signs of generational repetition, developed esteem, and found their voices.

It was a long road paved with an overwhelming amount of internal dialogue such as "How could he? Why am I not enough? How will I live? How will I manage?" "I'll never trust again." But these women discovered an inner strength they had never before experienced, and in that strength they found esteem; the skills for genuine emotional intimacy, joy, and laughter; and inner peace. The Serenity Prayer became the staple of their life.

God, grant me the serenity
To accept the things I cannot change, The
courage to change the things I can, And the
wisdom to know the difference.

Although others have walked before you, this is your very own unique journey. You are to be congratulated for coming this far, reading this book, and facing your truths. It takes courage, and you have it within you.

The journey of self-discovery will offer you many gifts. You don't have to live in the shadow of someone's addiction or be manipulated and controlled by anyone else's behavior. You can learn to trust yourself—in essence, to listen and trust "your worms." This is your opportunity to learn about healthy boundaries, who is responsible for what, and what gives you a sense of safety. As you begin this journey, remember that it's all about honoring and respecting yourself. You can move from immobilization or reactivity to a life of hope, greater esteem, and greater choices. While no one can walk the road of recovery for you, there are others who have traveled a similar path who will assist you. When all seems dark, there are people out their who will shine the light that helps you to continue moving forward. As you begin your healing, you will find an inner strength that allows you to transcend the pain; you will learn to trust in yourself and find meaning from the experience.

You don't have to come to recovery knowing what you want for your relationship; you don't even have to be in a relationship. You don't have to come eagerly. In truth, I suspect that you will come haltingly; you will be angry, sad, and very confused. I simply encourage you to come and begin your journey.

We are sisters and together we heal.

Reflective Thoughts and Questions

- Underline or highlight the parts of the women's stories with which you identify.

- What can you take from the different women to inspire your own healing and recovery process?

- What you are willing to do for yourself in your healing process? Be specific.

- What gifts are you already aware of receiving in this healing process?

- What potential gifts do you see for yourself as you continue?

- What was important for you to learn in this chapter?

Helpful Resources

Professionals Trained in Sexual Betrayal, Compulsive Sexual Behaviors, and Partner Trauma

- Association of Partners of Sex Addicts Trauma Specialists (APSATS)
  www.apsats.org

- International Institute for Trauma and Addiction Professionals (IITAP)
  www.iitap.com

- Society for the Advancement of Sexual Health (SASH)
  www.sash.net

- Rio Retreat Center, Intimate Treason Workshops
  www.rioretreatcenter.com

- Sex Help
  www.sexhelp.com

- Faithful and True
  www.faithfulandtrue.com

Trauma Resources

- Eye Movement Desensitization and Reprocessing (EMDR)
  www.emdria.org

- Sensorimotor Psychotherapy Institute
  www.sensorimotorpsychotherapy.org

- Somatic Experiencing Trauma Institute
  Find a certified Somatic Experiencing Practitioner (SEP)
  www.traumahealing.org

- Dialectical Behavior Therapy (DBT)
  www.behavioraltech.org

Twelve-Step Support Groups Dedicated to Helping Partners

- Partners of Sex Addicts (POSA)
  www.posarc.com

- Infidelity Survivors Anonymous (ISA)
  www.isurvivors.org

- Co-Dependents Anonymous International (CODA)
  www.coda.org

- Co-Dependents of Sex Addicts (COSA)
  www.cosa-recovery.org

- S-Anon
  www.sanon.org

- Al-Anon
  www.alanon.org

- Recovering Couples Anonymous (RCA)
  www.recovering-couples.org

- Sex and Love Addicts Anonymous (SLAA)
  www.slaafws.org

Twelve-Step Programs Dedicated to Helping Those with Compulsive Sexual Behaviors

- Sex Addicts Anonymous (SAA)
  www.saa-recovery.org

- Sexaholics Anonymous (SA)
  www.sa.org

- Sexual Compulsives Anonymous (SCA)
  www.sca-recovery.org

- Sex and Love Addicts Anonymous (SLAA)
  www.slaafws.org

Twelve-Step Programs Dedicated to Substance Use Disorders

- Alcoholics Anonymous (A twelve-step program of recovery
  from alcohol abuse)
  www.alcoholics-anonymous.org

- Narcotics Anonymous (A twelve-step program for
  recovery from drug addiction)
  www.na.org

Also Available by Claudia Black

Claudia Black Library CDs/DVDs

A Time for Healing
CD—705105051130

Addiction in the Family
DVD—705105051932

Anger
DVD—705105051833

Breaking the Silence
DVD

Children of Denial
DVD—705105052137

Compulsive Relationships
DVD

Double Jeopardy
DVD—705105052236

Emotional Baggage
CD—705105051239

**Healing from Childhood
Sexual Abuse**
DVD

History of Addiction
DVD

Imageries
CD—705105051338

Issues of Recovery
DVD—705105052335

Legacy of Addiction, The
DVD—705105052434

Letting Go Imageries
CD—705105051437

Putting the Past Behind
CD—705105051536

Relapse
DVD—705105052533

Relationship Building
DVD

Relationship Styles
DVD

Trauma in the Addicted Family
CD—705105051635

Triggering Effect
DVD—705105052632

Triggers
CD—705105051734

What Do I Say to My Kids
DVD—705105052731

Claudia Black Library Books

Changing Course
9781949481129

Anger Strategies
0910223300

Depression Strategies
0910223289

Family Strategies
0910223297

A Hole in the Sidewalk
9781942094739

Intimate Treason
9781936290932

It Will Never Happen to Me
9781949481105

My Dad Loves Me, My Dad Has a Disease
9781942094753

Relapse Toolkit
0910223262

Repeat after Me
9781942094777

Straight Talk
9781949481143

The Truth Begins with You
9781936290611

Unspoken Legacy
9781942094562